Mind Crisis

a story of loss and awakening

E. Patrick Hanavan III

Published by EPH3 Press
208 Arrowhead Ct, Winter Springs, Florida 32708

Some names and identifying details have been changed to protect the privacy of individuals.

Dedication

To the memory of my son, Ernest Patrick Hanavan IV.

Son, brother, grandson, nephew, cousin, friend, co-worker.

Fisherman, surfer, car lover, skateboarder, gamer, nature lover.

Beautiful, spiritual, loving soul.

an introduction

I believe everyone has a book in them, because we all have different experiences and so many different stories we could tell. Many years ago, after our daughter, Christine, graduated from college with a degree in creative writing, we set out to write a book together. Long story short, after much progress and several drafts, it was set aside because other interests came up for Christine. And I went back to my regular routine, believing that the book that was in me would never be published.

Fast forward to the summer of 2019, and I was in a two day onsite/offsite with the executive team from my company and our Leadership Coach and Organizational Psychologist, Dr. Laura, and I shared my belief that everyone has a book in them. But the book I was hinting at this time was very different from the fantasy one that Christine and I had started. After sleeping on it and having considered the potential benefits compared to the difficulties I would face, I committed to at least try. I decided to write every morning until I reached the point where I was exhausted emotionally, or I had exhausted what I wished to share.

And so, it begins....

Table of Contents

Why me? ______ *1*

woulda, coulda, shoulda ______ *3*

Confidence ______ *6*

TRAGIC ______ *10*

Fear ______ *15*

Get Lost ______ *19*

Nature ______ *24*

The Wind ______ *26*

Escape ______ *29*

Quirks ______ *34*

Showing up ______ *37*

World Cup ______ *42*

Hermit Crab ______ *46*

Church ______ *52*

CONSEQUENCES ______ *56*

Music ______ *59*

Alone ______ *63*

Holidays ______ *67*

Beacon ______ *71*

Selling ______ *76*

PICK UP THE PIECES — *82*
"Best Day of My Life" — *90*
RADIOACTIVE — *95*
Accelerate — *99*
Eye on the Goal — *102*
Denial — *105*
Steer — *109*
Salamander — *113*
Elephant — *117*
CHECK-IN — *121*
HOW — *127*
Epilogue — *130*
About the Author — *133*
Appreciation — *135*
Acknowledgements — *137*

Mind Crisis

a story of loss and awakening

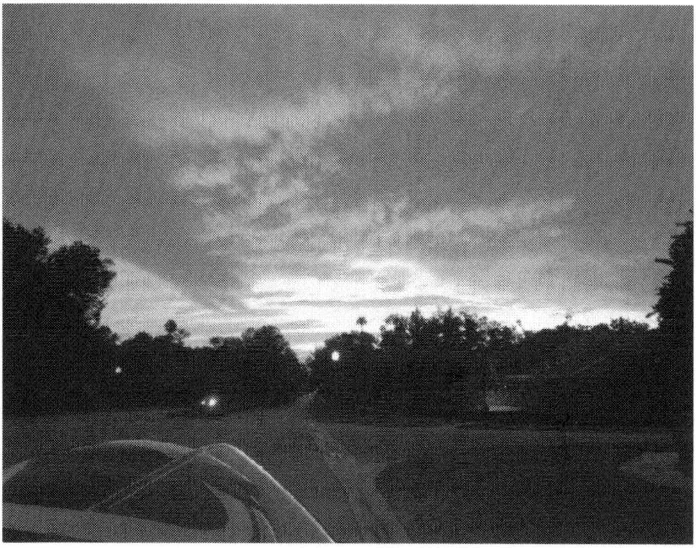

Why me?

We are all on this journey called *life*, but many of us struggle with what seems to be the simple things.

Whether we know it or not, we are surrounded by people who are struggling.

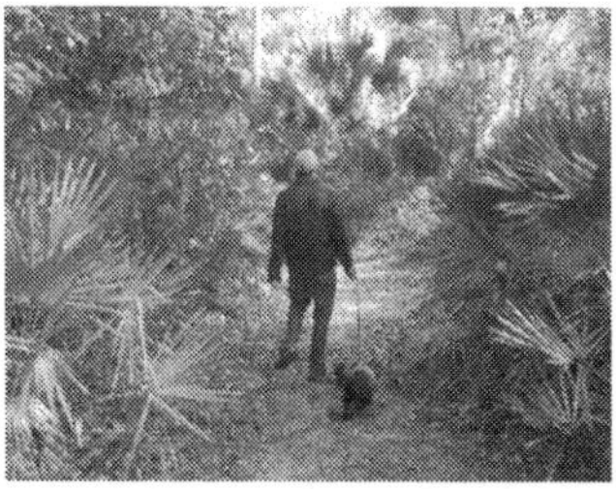

I was blessed to have had a son, Patrick IV, and I wanted desperately for him to be happy and enjoy life. But life seemed to always be difficult for him. He found the most pleasure and tranquility in communing with nature, whether it was from taking long nature walks, going fishing, or surfing at the beach. He had many friends who went fishing or surfing with him regularly, but he would also go out on his own often. He would ask to go on Can-Am Spyder motorcycle rides with me, and we enjoyed those times together very much.

But the good feelings he got from being out in nature were offset by bad thoughts and feelings that tormented him. Ultimately, the torments won out and he took his own life on August 7, 2015, a couple months shy of his 31st birthday.

If we don't deal with the stigma around mental health, we will continue losing loved ones and friends. Check the headlines. The suicide rate has increased 33% since 1999.

And it's alarming to see the number of young people committing suicide lately. I can't recall the last time I went a week without hearing of someone taking their own life, whether it was someone famous or a family member, a friend or a friend of a friend. At what point will we as a society realize that there's a suicide crisis happening? How should we react to the crisis that is claiming so many lives, especially those of our children?

> How would it feel to embrace those who are hurting, and support them however we can?
>
> How would it feel if we turn our backs on those in pain, and instead have to attend their funeral?

In this book, I intend to share thoughts and memories that I hope will strike a chord with people who have family members or friends who are struggling with mental health issues. It is my sincere hope that the deeply personal sharing I intend to do will be beneficial to others. Selfishly, I am also hoping that I can work through some of my own emotional aches and pains.

As much as I tell people that "I'm ok," sometimes it's just a platitude so they will not worry. Was that a cry for help? I don't believe so. The sad fact is that you never know what people are thinking or how they are feeling.

For me, I'm ok. Really.

At least that's the story I'm telling myself.

woulda, coulda, shoulda

I embarked on this journey focused on a goal of helping people like me, who have loved ones and friends that struggle with life, and are depressed and teeter on the edge of suicide. My son, Patrick, rode the emotional rollercoaster for many, many years before finally choosing to end his pain and struggles. Being there with him, and for him through much of that was extremely difficult at times; I felt like an emotional crutch that he had to lean on regularly. While it meant that I got to spend time with him, many times we were simply together but not verbally communicating. It seemed enough at the time, but I often thought that I should do more.

Patrick has been gone now for nearly four years, and the trap that I fall into still is what I call *woulda, coulda, shoulda* where I drag myself back in time to find fault with what I *would have* or *could have* or *should have* done differently so that my son would still be with me today. Since I can't change the past, it's a futile effort going there mentally and ultimately it only makes me feel worse. Within days of Patrick's death, Lydia's (my wife) psychiatrist, Dr. Carol, told us that we had done everything we could have to help him, and from her perspective, we had actually done far more than typical parents would have done in a similar situation. Although it was meant to help us feel better, it brought memories into focus and I couldn't help but question choices I had made about how I communicated with my son.

> Two days before he killed himself, Patrick came to our house in the evening. I could tell immediately that it was going to be one of those visits where

> he was feeling really bad, but he wasn't prepared to talk about it. In my opinion, most of his pain was self-inflicted in that he would make mountains out of molehills. Something or someone in his life would upset him and he would blow the situation out of proportion, grinding his wheels on it over and over and over. In these situations, I would often try to get him to see the situation in a different light, stressing that I doubted that the other person did the thing intentionally to hurt him. But such was his mental outlook that he would rarely listen to me. On this particular evening, I sensed that something was bothering him a great deal, more than usual, but he would not talk about it. At the time I was certain that it was something related to work. Because he seemed to be struggling so much with it, I made yet another attempt to convince him to seek out professional help. I encouraged him to see Lydia's psychiatrist or someone else and I told him that I desperately wanted him to feel better and I would pay for it and he needn't pay me back. I said that I wanted the best outcome for him. Sadly, that was the last conversation I had with Patrick. I know now that the thing he was struggling with was his decision to end his own life. It wasn't work. I was wrong, and I didn't recognize the signs. If I *could have* detected that his situation and mood were different than other times, I *would have* tried something different. I *should have* picked up that this time was different.

The *woulda, coulda, shoulda* thoughts are a slippery slope that can drag me back to the past, having me churn over memories that can't be changed. Letting myself slide back there doesn't do anything to help my own state of mind and mental health. Actually, it does quite the opposite. Another rather trite way I attempt to stay away from the slippery slope is to say "Look forward, not backward." I have to remind myself of this at times, and I say it often to Lydia and Christine, especially when we are reminded of Patrick and the difficult times we shared.

Confidence

As I was waking up this morning, I had a single word on my mind, CONFIDENCE. I find that I experience moments of clarity and/or creativity when I'm part way between a dream and awake state. This morning was one of those moments. As I have started working on my book in earnest, I'm trying to be more mindful of these opportunities and glimpses of insight into my own psyche.

Confidence

Why did my mind go there? As I was coming more fully awake, images of situations and memories were coming into focus. I have always struggled with a lack of confidence.

Confidence in my own abilities.

Confidence that I can accomplish what I set out to do.

Confidence that I am worthy of my wife's love for me.

Confidence in relationships with family.

Confidence that I'm a good father.

Confidence that I can provide for my family.

Confidence that I will succeed.

Confidence that I will satisfy co-workers.

Why do I struggle with this? Do others share the same paralyzing fear of failure that I experience? Recently my coach said that she admired my courage. I can understand why she said that, because of the nature and extent of sharing and openness that I exhibited in leadership growth sessions we had at our office. I am usually not very open or vulnerable with people around me, be they family, friends or co-workers. I've always been very shy and reserved, and when I do open up I do so in a calculated and careful way. You can see a little more of me, but not the full picture usually. In recent weeks I have been practicing more openness and being more vulnerable, with less concern over how people will react to me.

I must say that I have found the experiment to be liberating. It's an experiment because it seems that I'm on a journey to be a new me. And with each new step down unfamiliar pathways, I am learning a bit more about myself. And, I'm finding new levels of confidence in my interactions with others.

While in that half-way dream state this morning, after thoughts about myself, my thoughts turned to Patrick. In many ways, he was very much like me.

> Patrick lacked confidence in his interactions with others. We would talk about difficult situations or difficult people and I would share observations or stories from my life in an effort to help him see how his own insecurities were affecting his perceptions. Such was the way his brain operated that he could understand what I was saying, but he would usually remain fixated on his own view.

Patrick had many good friends and seemed to have solid relationships with them although none of them knew the full extent of the pains he was dealing with. Although Patrick suffered from the same type of paralyzing fear of failure that I feel at times, he put on a great face.

After his death, one of his co-workers came to our house to drop off things that Patrick had left at his office. Yet again I heard comments like "I had no idea," "He didn't seem depressed," "I wish I knew" and "Patrick always raised my spirits." These kind of comments and sentiments reminded me of so many people's reactions when Robin Williams took his own life on August 11, 2014 nearly one year before Patrick's suicide.

In my experience, I find it rare that people will share mental health struggles with others. The stigma that still surrounds mental health is a key reason why Patrick didn't seek out professional help. He was petrified of how friends and co-workers would perceive him if they knew that he had mental health issues. He argued that he would have to take time off from work for regular doctor visits, and that meant he would have to tell people why he wasn't in the office. And so, he wouldn't do it and instead self-medicated with caffeine, nicotine and marijuana.

The number and frequency of suicides happening today is reaching crisis levels. Isn't it well past the time for us to shatter the stigma surrounding mental illness? If we don't, lives will continue being shattered when those with mental illness decide that they can't cope with it any longer.

TRAGIC

Ugh! Why did I have to wake up this morning with the word TRAGIC on my mind? Unlike some other mornings, I didn't transition slowly from a dream state to being awake, where the creativity I mentioned before seems to be the strongest for me. Not this morning. Today I woke up and with no thoughts about what I would write about today, the word TRAGIC came to my consciousness.

It's so obvious. Of course, when someone commits suicide it's a tragedy. The Merriam-Webster dictionary defines tragic as:

> **1a:** regrettably serious or unpleasant :
>
> DEPLORABLE, LAMENTABLE
>
> a *tragic* mistake
>
> **b:** marked by a sense of tragedy
>
> **2:** of, marked by, or expressive of tragedy
>
> the *tragic* significance of the atomic bomb— H. S. Truman
>
> **3a:** dealing with or treated in
>
> tragedy the *tragic* hero
>
> **b:** appropriate to or typical of tragedy
>
> Examples of *tragic* in a Sentence
> Their deaths were *tragic* and untimely.
> They both died in a *tragic* car accident.

Patrick's death shocked family and friends, but it wasn't a shock to me, Lydia or Christine. We had been dealing with Patrick's depression and severe mood swings for many years, and I had had a foreshadowing of his death several years earlier.

> In the spring of 2011, I was out on a weekday afternoon riding my Can-Am Spyder in the Ocala National Forest area near Altoona, Florida. I needed to take a break from work because of all of the business travel I had been doing. Taking the Spyder out was a good way to clear my head and I was nearing the halfway point of my planned route when Patrick called me. He would never call me just to chat. Either something was wrong, or he needed something from me. With no preamble, Patrick said "I want to buy a gun." When I heard those five words from him, a chill went down my back and I had a vivid premonition of his death. I saw him lying on the floor of the bathroom with a gunshot wound to the forehead. After coming back to my present situation, I immediately responded to Patrick that he couldn't have a gun. He wanted to argue with me, but I shut down the conversation saying that it wasn't a good time to talk as I was riding and that we would discuss it later.
>
> The fact was, Patrick didn't need my permission to buy a gun. He was in his late twenties at the time. Plus, being a gun owner myself it seemed hypocritical of me to try to stop him. And, I was also concerned about how it might damage our relationship. After a few minutes of riding and thinking it through some more, I called Patrick back and asked him "Why?" I figured that he

might want to go to the range sometimes, and we could do that without his owning a weapon. I would have never guessed his reasoning. Patrick was an avid fisherman, and he was always searching for new places to fish. Recently, he was going out to an area around Bethune Beach on the Indian River. He would go out there, park his car and hike to a spot where he would fish. And the area was known to have alligators. His logic for getting a handgun was for personal protection from alligators. I tried to argue that he shouldn't fish there if it was dangerous, but when Patrick got a notion like this into his head he would fixate on it. Instead of getting into a long debate as I was riding, we agreed to talk about it in person. Suffice it to say that Patrick convinced me of his sincerity and attention to gun safety such that I supported his decision to get a handgun. For a few years after that, everything was fine and he and I would go to the range together sometimes.

Fast forward a few years, and Patrick was very depressed again. This time it was from struggles he was having in college. He had a group project for one of his business classes and not all members of his team cared as much about the end result as he did. He fixated on the potential failure of the project and resulting bad grade he would get. Such was the depth of his worry over the situation that he even considered leaving college and joining the military.

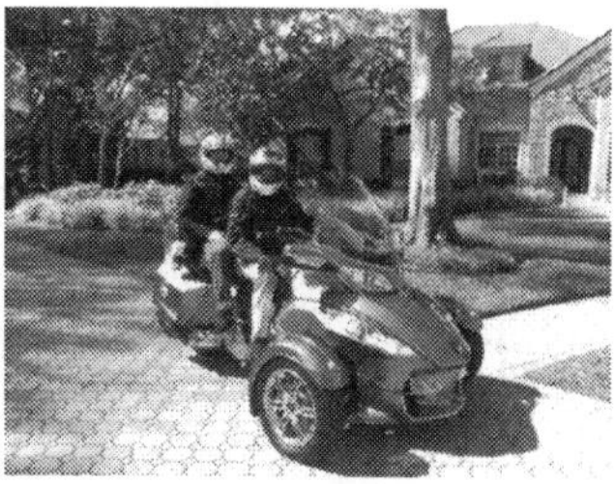

We went riding together on my Spyder soon after that conversation and we talked some about the situation while riding (using radios in our helmets). When we came home, I shared with him that I was extremely concerned about his state of mind, and I was particularly nervous about guns that he had at home. I was clear with him that I thought he might hurt himself and I asked if he would willingly give me the weapons for safe keeping. With no hesitation whatsoever, Patrick agreed adding that "I would never do that. Believe me."

I kept his weapons in my gun safe for well over a year. He graduated from the University of Central Florida (UCF) with a degree in Business Administration in August of 2012. He had taken a long road to get there, but he completed that journey and we were so very proud of him for sticking with it. After seeing him settle into a full-time job and believing his state of mind and mental health so much better than before, I started to worry a bit less about him. Seeing him happier and more settled, I returned his weapons when he asked and we started going back to the range.

Over the weeks and months prior to Patrick's suicide, although I was concerned about his state of mind my thoughts didn't return to the vision I had had years before.

Patrick had been very convincing when he told me "I would never do that." And I convinced myself that I needn't worry about that any more.

I could not have been more wrong. Three years later he would do that thing that he said he would never do. And I found him just like I had seen in my vision four years earlier. I had been able to intervene at a critical time. Once. Tragically, I only delayed the inevitable.

TRAGIC

Fear

This morning was different for a few reasons: 1) it's Saturday so I don't have time pressure to go into work, 2) I'm up earlier than usual because we're going Spyder riding this morning with friends to Crabby Joe's in Daytona Beach for brunch, 3) I do have time pressure because I need to finish getting ready for the ride, including topping up gas in the Spyder, and 4) I didn't wake up with a flash of inspiration for today's chapter.

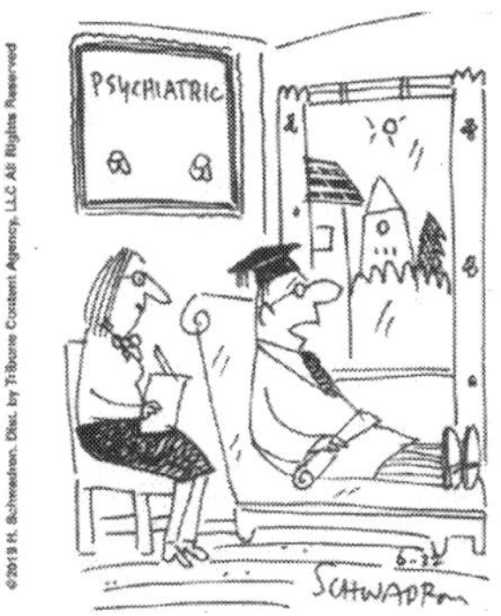

"I have this fear of the real world..."

Nevertheless, inspiration came to me in the form of a comic strip. For 20+ years part of my morning routine has been to read my favorite comics. I stopped subscribing to the newspaper ages ago when I realized that all I cared to read regularly was the comics page. I found an online way to subscribe to my favorites and I wake up every day with my favorite comic strips in my inbox. Harley Schwadron's *9 to 5* today was this. It summarizes Patrick's long journey through college, other than the visit to the psychiatrist.

> Patrick graduated from high school in 2003 and graduated from college in 2012. He changed his major area of study multiple times and attended three different colleges before earning his undergraduate degree. Fear was at the core of why it took him that long to finish.

Fear of failure.

Fear of responsibility.

Fear of life.

Fear of the real world.

I know this because he finally confided in me about what he had been doing. Because of his near crippling fear of failure, he would only take a handful of classes at a time and he would often drop a class if he wasn't confident of making an A in it. He failed out of UCF after his first semester there, losing his fully paid scholarship as a result. That first semester hit him really hard, largely because of the difficult course load that he took on and also because he felt totally lost in the faster pace, higher pressure, self-motivated environment of college. It was at this time that he retreated into self-medicating using marijuana.

After that first semester, Patrick came to Lydia and I begging for help because he knew how much the pot had taken him over. He was full of fear for his future and he asked for our help to get him back on track. He sought out professional help, but the psychologist recommended to us would not see him regularly unless he was already completely clean. It was a bad situation, a chicken-or-the-egg problem in that he needed help to get clean, but the psychologist would not even see him until he *was* clean. That totally demotivated Patrick and we couldn't even get him to seek out someone else. So, we tried our best to do everything we could to help him. We attempted to provide more structure for him, and I did random drug tests to keep him honest as he worked to get clean. I really didn't think it should be so difficult to get clean, but we didn't really know or understand the extent of Patrick's addiction and underlying mental state.

I was fearful for my son. Fearful for his future. Fearful that he would not complete college. Fearful that he wouldn't succeed professionally.

A year before Patrick graduated from college, he confided in me that he purposefully dragged out his time in college because he was afraid of independence and the responsibility of making a living for himself. He sincerely apologized because he knew that his behavior cost me money. I assured him that the money didn't matter and my only concern was for him to find happiness.

Hindsight is 20/20 and it's easy for me to say now that I was fearful for the wrong things. But as I have stated before, I don't want to *look backward* too much because that leads to *woulda, coulda, shoulda* thinking which will drag me down emotionally. I have to stop and remind myself because my mind can quickly go down the path of

I should have…

I could have…

I wish I had…

If I had only…

If I knew then what I know now…

The thing that tears me down the most emotionally these days is the fear that I have been a bad father. Family and friends have never said that to me, but it's what I see in the mirror sometimes. Thoughts of "Would Patrick still be with us if I had been a better father?" come to my mind sometimes. There is no way to answer that, and I believe that fixating on it leads down a path of self-destruction.

When a friend from college heard that I lost my son, he reached out to me saying:

> *I lost my eldest son almost 4 years ago. Your faith, family and friends will carry you in the coming days, weeks and years.*

His son "died suddenly" a few years prior (code for "died by suicide"), so he knew what I was going through. I really appreciated hearing those words of encouragement from him, partly because I knew that I wasn't alone.

A couple years later, I learned that my friend took his own life. It was crushing for me to hear that he also died at his own hand. He had lost his way, and evidently *faith, family and friends* weren't enough for him to carry on.

Get Lost

My first thought this morning when I woke up was "Get lost." It was directed to our tabby cat, Luke, who at the crack of dawn most mornings comes into our bedroom and starts yowling and running across our pillows to get Lydia or me to get up and feed him breakfast. Admittedly, this morning he was encouraged to start his morning ritual because my alarm had gone off at 6:15 AM. I have it set for that time so that I reserve enough time in the morning for writing before I jump in the shower and then head to work.

My alarm went off, and within seconds of that Luke yowled, jumped on the bed, ran across the pillows and landed on the night stand table next to my side of the bed. I really did not want to get up at 6:15 on a Sunday morning and my first thought of the day was directed to Luke. Using my best human-to-cat telepathy, I purposefully directed "Get lost" to Luke to get him to go away and leave us alone. What the hell. Nothing. Not even a single mew in recognition of "Message received." I guess I'd better go ahead and get up after all. At the very least, I have inspiration for something to write about today.

Get Lost

> When our kids were only a few years old, on weekends I would occasionally tell Lydia, "Let's get lost." I was referring to something I enjoyed doing where we would get into the car with the kids and we would drive westward from our home in San Antonio, Texas with the intention of seeing new sights in the Texas Hill Country. This was

long before GPS, Garmin, Google Maps, etc. and although we had a folded paper map of Texas in the car, I would not consult it. Fortunately for me, I have an excellent innate sense of direction, so I would very rarely ever get lost. As we trekked through the hill country, we would often discover nice, small towns we didn't know about along with scenic winding roads and restaurants we had never heard about. I thoroughly enjoyed these times and my family mostly tolerated it.

Some years later, my kids gave me a Hallmark card:

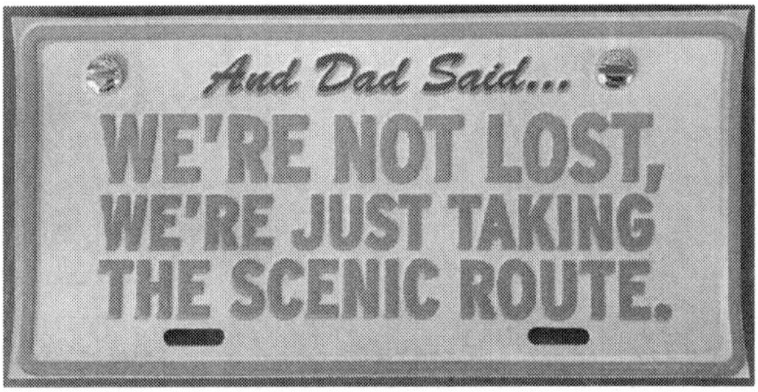

And inside "Thanks for showing us so much of the world."

I keep it on display in my home office because I still enjoy getting lost.

Fast forward a couple decades from those weekends of getting lost in the Texas Hill Country, and I would often ride my Can-Am Spyder on country roads all over Central Florida. While I would just drive around and take a random turn that I had not taken before, Patrick took it to a new level. After he had ridden with me several times, he started suggesting areas to explore and roads to take. Patrick was always searching for state parks we didn't know about, lakes and waterways where he could fish and new roads we hadn't ridden on yet. He became quite expert with doing online research, especially with Google Earth and Google Maps using the satellite view.

On Christmas day of 2013 we took our dog, Arwen, with us and went down the road a couple miles to a local park near our house. We had driven by that park too many times to count, but we had never ventured far into it. On this day, we decided to get lost in that park. We didn't actually get lost, but we explored the park fully, going all of the way through it to the other side until we had come upon the back sides of people's homes that are adjacent to it on its northern edge. Arwen was super excited to see new sights, but we did have to pick out sand spurs from her sweater when we returned to the car. Being in the calm setting of that park on Christmas day is one of my fondest memories of Patrick. He seemed to truly be at peace that day.

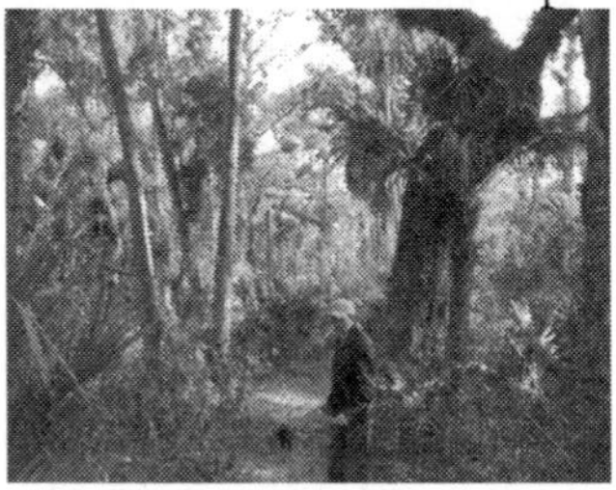

On Christmas day the following year, Patrick suggested taking the Spyder out for a ride and although surprised by the request, I agreed. After getting several miles away from our home, and on a road heading towards UCF, Patrick suggested taking a road we hadn't ridden on before. I did so without hesitation. After a few miles, Patrick came on the intercom and asked if I had seen the museum we just passed. "What museum?" was my reaction because I really hadn't seen anything. So, we doubled back to check it out. Out on North Tanner Road is a Vietnam War museum. I was surprised for several reasons. First, here was a museum that I had never heard about out in a rural area of Central Florida. Second, it's a museum to the Vietnam War and my father is a veteran of that war.

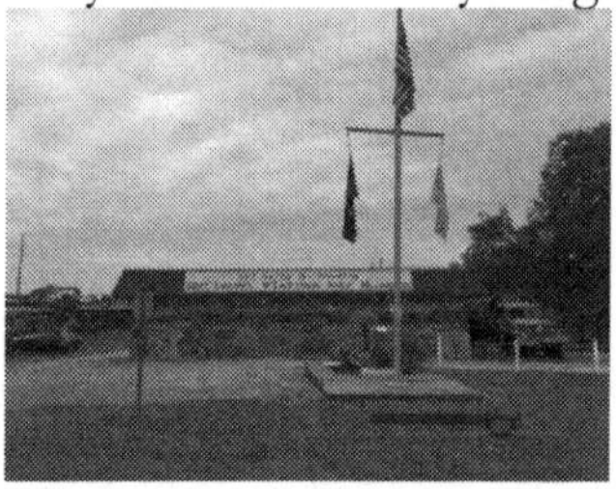

And thirdly, and most surprisingly, they had the front portion of a U.S. Air Force C-7A Caribou airplane on the property. My father was in the U.S. Air Force and flew Caribous in Vietnam. Mind blown! I sent a picture of it to my dad to see if he had any record of it. At the time, my father was the president of the Caribou Association and he was in the process of writing his books on the history of the Caribou in Vietnam. His group had records on every known surviving Caribou from that war, and Patrick and

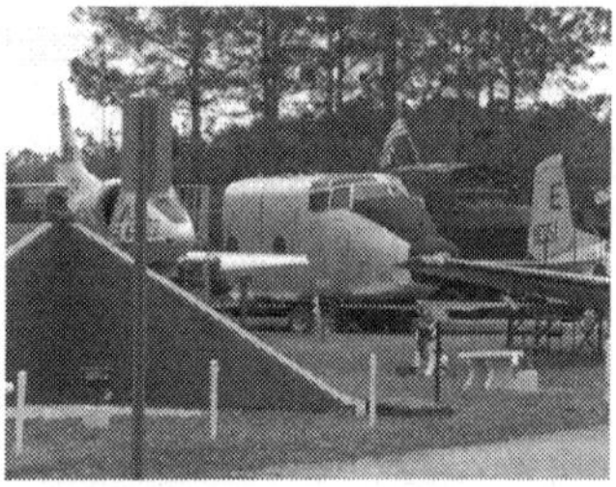

I might have found something that they did not know about.

Suffice it to say that with Patrick riding with me we discovered many roads and sights all over Central Florida. It became a goal for us to try to find something new when we ventured further away from areas and roadways that we already knew. We challenged ourselves to show the other something new that they hadn't seen yet. And I shared many of those new roads and sights with fellow Spyder riders when I organized group rides.

These days when I'm out riding by myself, I am still looking for those roads I haven't ridden yet. Sometimes as I ride, I calm myself down and search for the feeling I had when Patrick was riding with me. Although doing so can make me sad, it also helps me feel connected to him again. When I do find something new, or finally turn down a road I've gone past many times before, I often look up and point to the sky and say "This is for you, Patrick."

You never know what you will find when you get lost.

Nature

Sometimes when Patrick and I went out riding on the Spyder, he had a specific destination in mind. On those days, he was always taking me to a new park or spring that I hadn't seen before. I was really surprised how many of them were pretty close to where we lived.

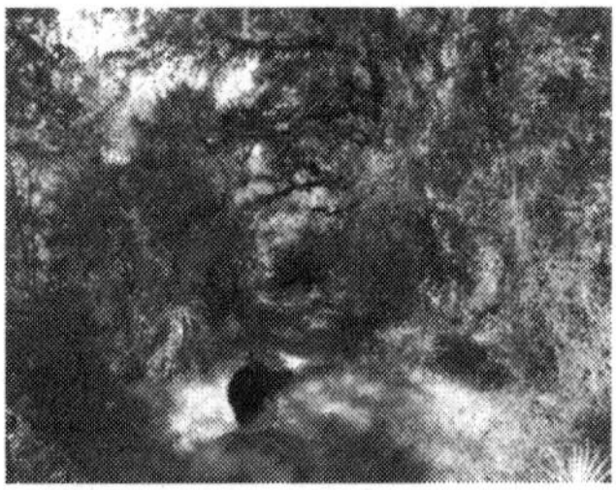

Patrick always seemed to be at peace most when he was out in nature. When we went on nature hikes together, he took great pleasure in showing me new trails, springs and waterways that I had not seen before. He would usually have checked out these places in advance, and then showed them to Lydia and me or just me if we were out on the Spyder. Sometimes we would take our dog with us too. He really enjoyed walking the dog on nature trails.

On the two weekends before he killed himself, Patrick took Lydia and me to see Smyrna Dunes Park, Cape Canaveral Seashores, Turtle Mound and Seminole Rest. These are all on the east coast of Central Florida, south of Daytona Beach. Although we had lived in Florida for nearly 30 years, we had never visited these sites. At the time, it seemed that Patrick was genuinely happy, but those blissful weekends were a stark contrast to how he was feeling at work during the week.

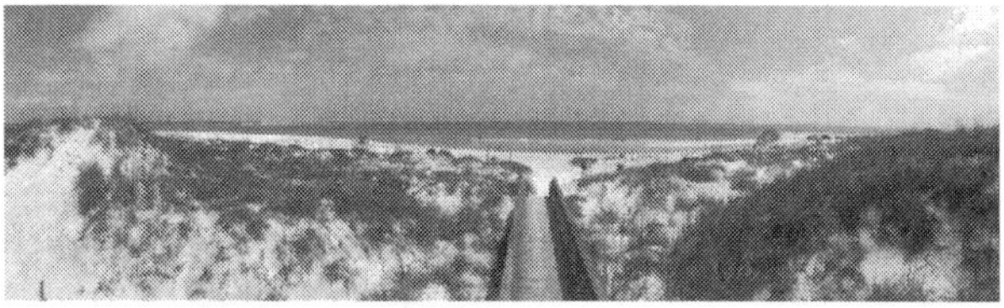

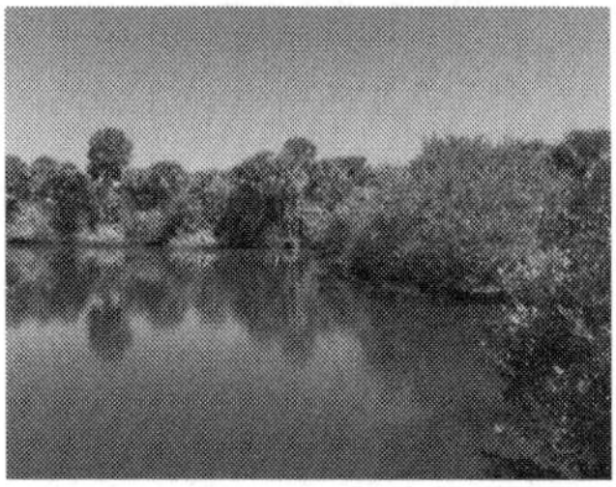

Other than pointing out things at these nature locations, he didn't talk a lot while we were there. He seemed to just be content to be. To me, it looked like he enjoyed the moments there. Being around nature seemed to have a calming effect for him but I can't know for certain.

On the second anniversary of his death, I asked Lydia to ride with me and we rode around to several of his favorite spots. I told Lydia that I wanted to see those sites again because I wanted to celebrate him and feel closer to him on that particular day. And I hoped that she would get something out of it too. Riding on those country roads and stopping at places like Gemini Springs, Green Springs, Little Big Econ Park and Mullet Lake Park were emotional for us because of the memories that were stirred up. Yes, it was emotional, but for me, I felt more inward calm than on the one-year anniversary of his death.

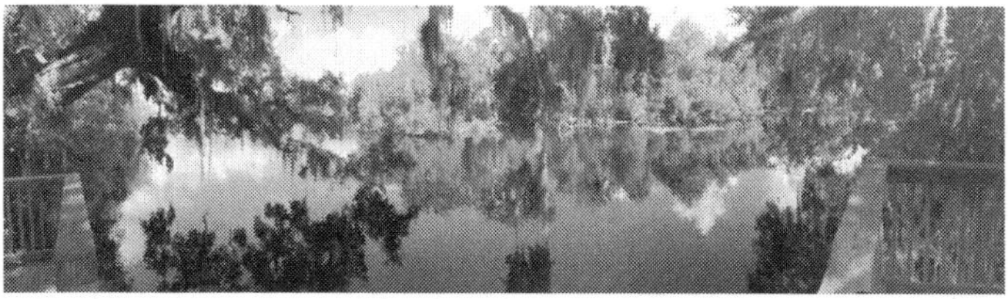

The Wind

Before my alarm went off this morning, I turned to my left side while asleep and was greeted with a face full of wind coming from a portable fan that Lydia had on her night stand table. I like wind, but not in my face while I'm trying to sleep. I lay there for a bit and woke up enough to start thinking about how the wind affects me. And Cat Steven's song *The Wind* came to me. His album *Teaser and the Firecat* was one of my favorites when I was in junior high school, and I used to play it over and over. The song opens with:

> *I listen to the wind, to the wind of my soul*
> *Where I'll end up, well, I think only God really knows*

The wind is a significant part of my life now, and it started when I got my first motorcycle. The first time I test rode one, I *got it.* I finally understood why people enjoy riding motorcycles. The combination of the openness while on the road, seeing the world around me while riding with no metal surrounding me, and having the wind in my face has a profound impact on my soul. For me, the experience is nothing short of amazing and it's why I often refer to the times I'm riding as *wind therapy*. Those first two lines from *The Wind* summarize my feelings while I'm riding. I often set out without any clear route or destination in mind, and I let the wind of my soul guide me.

A few mornings ago, I wrote about getting lost and taking new roads I haven't travelled before. Shortly after writing that, I set out on my Spyder with a goal of experiencing some new roads that morning. It has become more and more difficult to do, however, as I have already covered the majority of the roads around Central Florida over the past eight years. Have you ever approached an intersection that you've gone through many times before, and as you pass the road to the right you say to yourself "I wonder where that goes"? I used to do that a lot, but over recent years I have taken that road to the right to see where it leads me. Many roads turn out to be dead ends, but some go to places that are interesting and scenic.

Other than the obvious benefits of riding on new roads and seeing new sights, Patrick never told me why he enjoyed riding with me. I don't recall ever using the phrase *wind therapy* with him, but I could sense that he really appreciated the wind in the face feeling from riding.

One Saturday morning, Patrick and I were talking, and he started off by asking about whether I had ridden on some new roads he had discovered in his searches. He brought up a few, but I had already done those but then he mentioned Reed Ellis Road which is south of Osteen, Florida. It was one of those roads whose name I recognized because I had ridden past it many, many times but I had never turned down that road so I had no idea where it went. He continued by asking me if I had been to Green Springs Park before. I had never heard of that park. Ah ha! He was super excited to hear of a road and a park that I hadn't seen yet. We both exclaimed "Let's ride."

We took familiar roads getting to Reed Ellis Road, but it was an incredible sensation for me as I turned down that road. My senses almost tingled

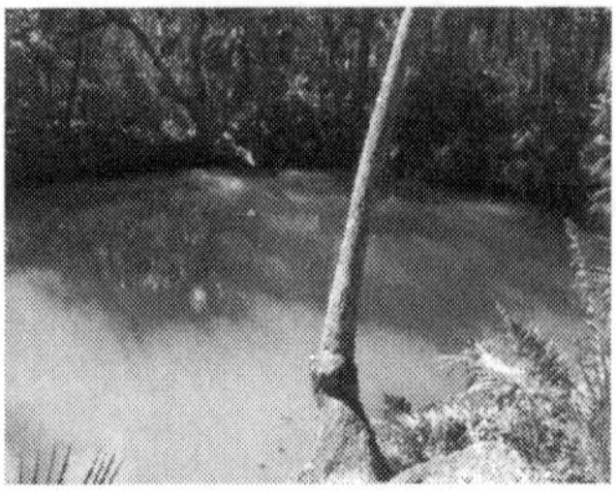

as I explored the new area. I recall a real sense of enjoyment and perhaps pride from Patrick as we rode together that morning. I turned west onto Enterprise Osteen Road to continue our journey, and subsequently turned into Green Springs Park when we arrived there. I parked the Spyder and Patrick showed me the trails, woods and springs of the park. We sat in silence for a long while enjoying the calm and quiet around the spring. The times that Patrick and I visited Green Springs Park were very special to me because I recalled his joy at sharing something new with me when we went there the first time. Patrick always seemed to be struggling with some sort of turmoil in his life (many times self-induced), but the *wind therapy* and being with nature helped him steady his emotional swings.

This morning I find myself wondering what it would be like to take new roads in interactions with other people. Perhaps it would lead to new understandings. Or a dead end. Either way, I think I would experience something new.

Time to put some *wind* in my face…

Escape

This morning's word appears to be *Escape* even though I tried to focus my thoughts on other subjects as I was waking up. Why was I trying to avoid writing about *Escape*? All I could come up with was that it was obvious and rather cliché, especially with respect to my son. I feared that there wasn't anything new or interesting to share with an examination of what *Escape* means to me.

Nevertheless, I decided to stick to my convictions for the process I am following for my daily reflections. And so *Escape* it is.

Why was escape foremost in my mind this morning? I can think of a few reasons why. Upon the conclusion of *The Big Bang Theory* television series earlier this year, I decided to go back and watch the full story arc again. Last night I watched the episode *The Intimacy Acceleration*, which included a scene where Leonard, Amy, Raj and Emily went to an escape room where they solved the puzzles in the room lightning fast and escaped in less than ten minutes. And a couple months ago, my company went to The Escape Game Orlando on International Drive one afternoon. Six teams did six different rooms of various levels of difficulty. My group was the only one that didn't escape; we ran out of time before we solved the last few clues. I hate losing, but we were able to rationalize the loss because we did the most difficult room which is designed for an 85% failure rate.

Why else is *escape* on my mind this morning? Curiously enough, before waking up fully I was dreaming about a strange situation where I was at some conference or large business meeting at a resort type location and I couldn't get away from it after it concluded. The conference was in the process of winding down, and somehow my attempts to leave kept getting thwarted. I spent the rest of the dream trying in vain to escape from the resort. I distinctly remember feeling trapped and unable to alter the outcome of what was happening to me. Thankfully, I woke up a few minutes before my alarm would usually go off. And I had *escape* on my mind.

Contemplating *escape* made me think about how it was something that Patrick dealt with.

> Patrick would escape from his day-to-day issues by going to the beach, taking nature walks, fishing or riding with me on the Spyder.

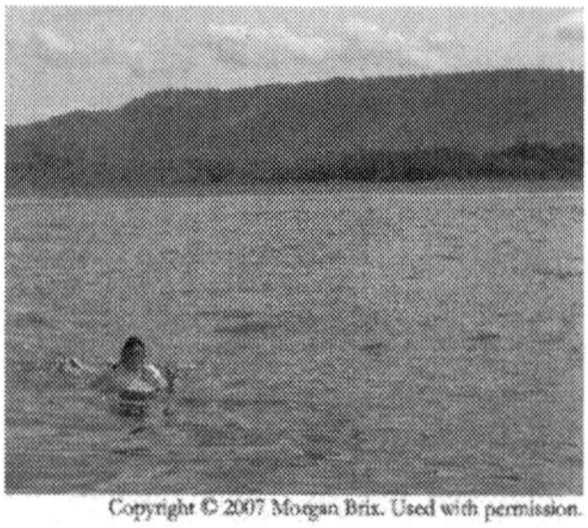

> I wanted desperately for Patrick to find happiness or at least acceptance of life so that he would stop having such severe mood swings. I was happy for him whenever I saw him head out to go surfing or fishing. And most times I was happy to jump on the Spyder and go riding with him. Clearly, those activities were an escape for him from whatever demons were plaguing him.

> After his death, and with repeated thoughts of *why?*, I came up with my own interpretation of why he killed himself. It's my interpretation because

he didn't tell us why. And I can tell you that the combination of *woulda, coulda, shoulda* and *why?* can be debilitating. On multiple occasions, I have had to pull myself back from the edge of the wormhole that those thoughts accelerate one towards. And, I have had to help pull others back, too, be they family or friends.

I really wanted to know why, and when I got his laptop back from the police I went digging for answers. After many hours of searching, I can tell you that I found nothing on it. There was no goodbye letter, or explanation of why he did it. There was no evidence of options he considered for ending his life, either. And Patrick was so worried about how other people viewed him that he didn't have any social media accounts. He wasn't happy with me if I shared pictures of him on Facebook or my websites. And on a few occasions, he would go so far as to ask me to remove them.

Across his laptop and cellphone, I did find a massive collection of pictures from him fishing. It was his favorite escape and he documented his fishing escapades very well. But, I was left with no answer from him as to *why?*

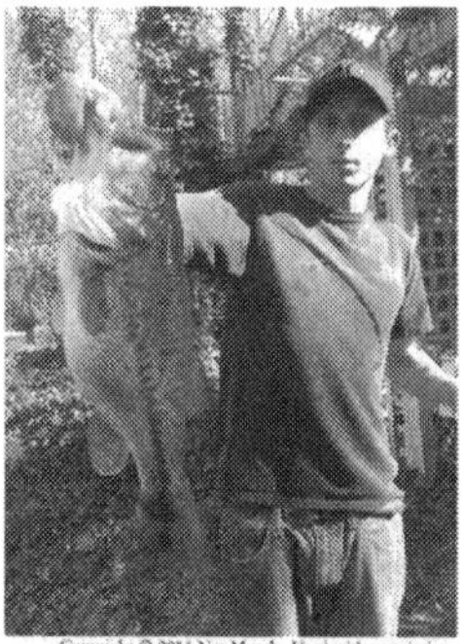

I honestly didn't need to find that last note to Mom and Dad. I already

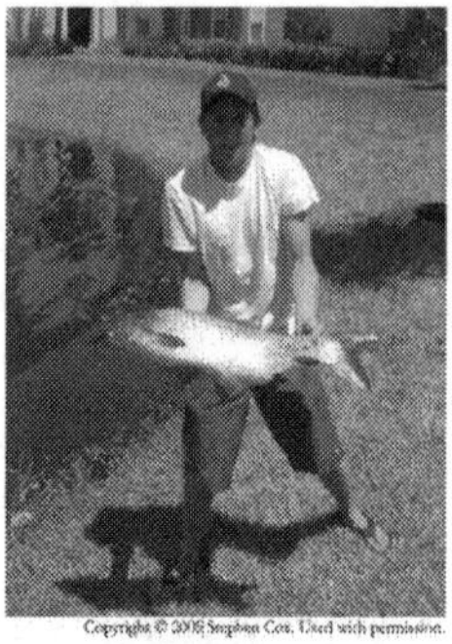

knew why. Patrick had struggled with life for YEARS. When he was seven years old, he took a pair of scissors to Lydia and asked her to kill him. That was the first sign of his struggles and dark thoughts. And while dating "blondie" during high school, who herself had serious emotional issues, he considered hurting himself. He didn't do anything to himself then, but he carved a hole in the top of his desk to channel his frustrations.

The bottom line is that he was done with life. His struggles coping with interpersonal interactions along with him blowing situations out of proportion combined to drag him down into depression, and he would stay there for long stretches of time. Yes, his mood would swing more positive with the activities I mentioned earlier but even his highest highs would be offset by incredible lows.

Since Patrick's death, I have cycled through thoughts of *why?* Over and over, mostly when visiting his gravesite. But I always return to the same answer. Patrick couldn't find happiness and contentment, and instead was convinced that he would never feel better and so he took the ultimate…

...escape.

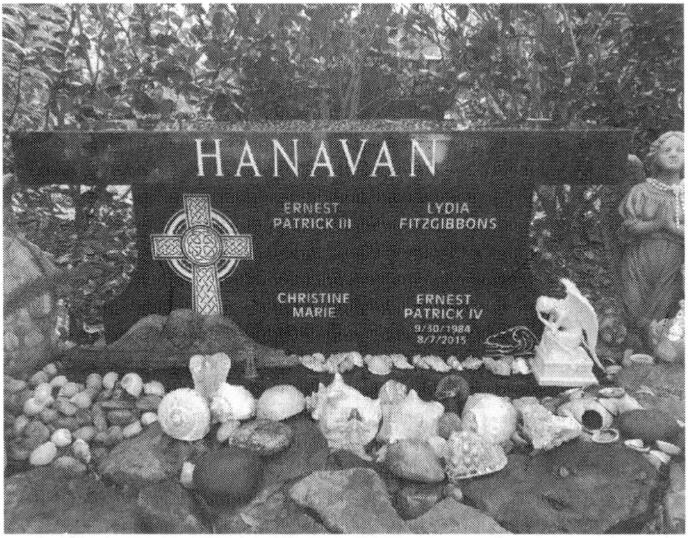
HANAVAN
ERNEST
PATRICK III
LYDIA
FITZGIBBONS
CHRISTINE
MARIE
ERNEST
PATRICK IV
9/30/1984
8/7/2015

Quirks

Nope. I'm not getting up at 5:50 AM today, Luke. For some odd reason this morning, Luke decided to start his morning *time to wake up Pat* ritual (yowling and running across the pillows) even earlier than usual. The sun was definitely not up yet. Groan. Not this morning! I got out of bed briefly and banished Luke and his brother, Han, from the master bedroom. Curiously enough, their sister, Leia (our rat terrier dog) wasn't stirring very much yet. As I got back into bed, I glanced over at Leia to see how she was reacting to the situation. She had eyes on me, and as I settled back into bed, she moved to rest her chin on my leg, which is a cute quirk of hers.

This morning, I wasn't ready to get up twenty minutes earlier than usual, so I tried to go back to sleep. But that hardly ever works for me. Once I'm awake, that's it. I laid in bed for a few minutes and thought about the oddities, or *quirks*, that our pets exhibit. Our pets are full of them.

It seemed doubly odd to me that the word *quirks* might be the inspiration for today's writing. I'm sure I have at least some quirks but I'm not sure what they are. And I suppose we all have quirks to some degree, right? Patrick had quite a few…

> He never wanted to wear shirts with advertising on them. It was a waste of money for me to bring back t-shirts from places I had visited on business trips because he would never wear them. For his birthday one year, I gave Patrick a nice collared shirt with a BMW logo but he never wore it.

Patrick was really paranoid about the potential for being spied upon. Friends and friends of friends had shared stories with him where they believed issues they had with local or federal government came from those agencies spying on them. He resisted the idea of getting a credit card because of paranoia that government or business could track his behavior, but he would still use his debit card for purchases. And as I've shared before, he didn't want pictures of himself on the internet for similar reasons.

He would lose his wallet and/or debit card frequently. This frustrated me immensely because it would happen so often, sometimes three or four times in a single year.

He wore flip-flops or sandals most of the time. Although I noticed this, it didn't bother me at all. My brother, Mike, also noticed it and thought it odd enough that he remarked regularly about it to Patrick. Patrick was so self-conscious that this would really bother him and it actually damaged their relationship.

Until the last couple years of his life, Patrick would not wear a watch. I really don't know why he changed his position on that.

He was really hard on his glasses and would regularly lose or break them.

After looking back over this list of what I thought were *quirks* that Patrick had, I think some of them were more serious. But I would cause him more grief any time I tried to probe into one of those subjects with him. I wanted to help him, but he didn't seem to want my help. Eventually, I learned that I should let things be because the alternative made him feel worse, not better.

And so, I did nothing to help him with these. And I felt helpless knowing that Patrick was in pain and also knowing that I could not do anything.

Showing up

How are we *showing up* in our daily interactions with family, friends and co-workers? What are we communicating to others about how we are feeling, and how we are handling life's journey? Whether we are aware of it, or not, we are communicating to others even when we're not talking, telegraphing a variety of emotions about how we are doing.

I'd like to think that I'm pretty good at "reading people," getting a sense of how they are doing simply from their body english and facial expressions. The fact is, most of us are not very good actors and we have little control over our own face when it comes to hiding our emotions. And even if we do, we slip at times and our true self is there for the world to see.

> "Are you ok, Pat?" – brother-in-law, Pete
>
> Oops! That happened yesterday evening while we were visiting Lydia's family in Georgia to celebrate her dad's 90th birthday. We had finished dinner and a few of us were in the living room together. I sat down at one side of the room, separate from anyone else.
>
> As I sat alone in my in-law's living room, I was overwhelmed all of a sudden with a feeling of isolation and being alone even though there were about twenty people in the house. I even noticed how I was at one end of the room while Pete and a few others were on the opposite side of the room. And I wondered why that was. Had I

deliberately isolated myself from everyone else? Since I was alone with my thoughts, I did something I had not done before – I started thinking about my writing outside of the morning ritual I do. I did a bit of a mental inventory of where I was at in the process so far and I thought about how I needed to go back and edit earlier content. That led to recalling some of the more difficult memories of Patrick I had shared thus far. And then, "Are you ok, Pat?"

In my reverie, I had inadvertently dropped my defenses and even though I wasn't saying anything with my mouth, I was clearly communicating my emotions, otherwise Pete would not have picked up on them. And unlike most people, I have acted (part time and non-professional), and I am usually in control of how I present myself non-verbally. Oops! On this occasion I had lost focus and my true self and feelings were visible for others to see.

Patrick had never acted in plays in school but he was a very good actor. I say that because he fooled nearly everyone all of his life. He was in pain and tormented by his own imagination and yet he hid that so very well. But, he also regularly avoided larger family gatherings and it was extremely rare that he would travel to visit either grandparents. The last time he did participate in a family gathering was for Lydia's dad's 85th birthday five years ago. I was quite surprised that he went with us, and he seemed to genuinely enjoy seeing everyone again.

Some years prior to that, we had reservations to spend several days with my parents and siblings in the Texas Hill Country, at a B&B outside Fredericksburg. We were going to gather together there around Easter; it was Lydia's suggestion to do that instead of getting together over Christmas which was typical for my family. I grew increasingly nervous leading up to that trip because it was a common occurrence for Patrick to cancel at the last minute. Most times he seemed to do it because something better came along, and he didn't seem to care that he had made a commitment to others. His pattern of cancellations was extremely frustrating to me. And sure enough, one day Lydia told me that Patrick could not go to Texas. She went on to say that we should not go. I was angry at first about the notion of cancelling, but then it was clear that Patrick was experiencing one of those very dark times in his life. We were extremely concerned about his state of mind and knew that we needed to surround him with love and support.

I called my dad and let him know that we could not make it. And for the first time ever, I let him in on the secret that Patrick had mental health issues. I asked that he keep that to himself as Patrick would be mortified if everyone in the family knew of his issues. I called the B&B to cancel, and instead of making up an excuse I explained that my son was dealing with very bad depression and we just could not make the trip. I asked for them to keep our deposit and we would return another time. The woman on the other end of the phone was very understanding because of mental health illness in her own family, and we ended up having a long conversation that helped us both.

I believe I now understand some of the contributing factors for why Patrick would cancel out of family gatherings regularly. And the main factor was *fear.* He was fearful of dealing with questions like…

Why are you taking so long in college?

Are you dating anyone now? No? When was the last time?

Why do you go surfing so much? Are you becoming a beach bum?

Why do you wear flip-flops all of the time?

Why don't we see you more?

What do you want to do when you graduate from college?

You lost your wallet again?

Patrick did not want to deal with the questions and the criticism that would come. As a result, family had no idea of what Patrick was struggling with. In those instances of him not being able to deal with the situation, he would simply not show up.

> On the surface, it seemed that he cared more about his friends than his family because he would spend time with the former and not the latter. That is definitely not true, but because of his state of mind he couldn't afford to be around family because it would only make him feel worse, not better.

I thought about *showing up* this morning primarily because of Pete checking up on me last night. He went on to say "You looked forlorn." Double oops! I had *really* let down my defenses for him to read that from me.

As I said before, most of us are not very good actors and we are regularly subconsciously communicating our emotions, feelings and state of mind to people around us. I mention this to encourage you to pay attention to those forms of communication, and check on people like how Pete did with me last night. A simple "Are you ok?" is an invitation to connect on an emotional level. And if someone is open enough to share their situation and pains with you, there's an opportunity for you to help them.

I implore you to pay attention to how others are *showing up* with you.

World Cup

Yesterday was the 2019 quarter final match between the U.S. and French Women World Cup teams. I started watching it last night after we returned home from Georgia in the afternoon. It was great to see the U.S. women beat the French team to advance to the semi-final round of the World Cup.

One of the best times in Patrick's life was the last championship match at the end of the time he played co-ed recreational soccer during his middle school years. The back story for that game is important to know, though.

Patrick played soccer for several years when he was in elementary school, and I was an assistant coach for his team. He played different defensive positions and he was a pretty good goal keeper, which is a stressful position to play. After a few years, the league that he was playing in folded and he didn't play for a semester because we had difficulty finding another league. Around this same time, we bought a new house and Patrick re-connected with someone he had known years earlier in school. The boy and his brother played soccer in a co-ed recreational league we didn't know about. There were less than ten teams in the league, but practices and games were nearby.

The most significant influence on the team came from Coach Leo who was an All-American goal keeper in college. He and I coached the team and we went from last place to first place in our first year. We won three straight championships and the kids were having a great time together! At the beginning of our fourth year, Coach Jack showed up with a team of "ringers" who also played in select teams in the area. We lost a few games during the regular season to them - our first losses in three years. The championship game for that season was between our two teams.

During the warm-up to our fourth consecutive championship game, our kids were distraught, convinced that we would lose, and someone even suggested walking off the field before kick-off as a final protest against the team of "ringers." Coach Leo and I argued that we would not do that. And Coach Leo dug back in his playbook and made an inspiring speech to the team that we *could* beat them. It was all about playing smart and using the fundamentals that they had learned during all of our practices. Coach Leo told the team that we would only play defense. We would strive for a 0-0 tie game, which given the makeup of Coach Jack's team would be a moral victory for us. The kids considered what Leo was asking of them, and they got excited at the possibility of frustrating Coach Jack's team.

At half-time, we were tied 0-0 and Coach Jack and his team were clearly confused because we did nothing but focus on defense. Patrick and his team mates had made some great defensive plays. They seemed to be playing on a whole new level, and it was an amazing thing to witness. Coach Leo turned to me at half-time and said "We can actually win this." What? I really didn't understand how we could win when we weren't even trying to mount an offense. He told the team to look for an opportunity for a break-away that the other team would not expect. There was excitement and hope in the kids' eyes now, unlike before the game started. They were doing exactly what we wanted them to do, and now they saw the potential to actually beat the unbeatable team.

During the second half, our team continued playing excellent defense. We stuck with the same goal keeper (our best) and he was on fire! I don't recall how many saves he made, but some of them seemed miraculous. We tried a couple breakaways, but those failed. With about ten minutes left in the game, the opportunity for another breakaway happened. A couple of our players drove into the opponent's side leaving Coach Jack's select players in the dust at first. As their defense caught up, a critical on-side pass was completed and our first shot on goal was attempted. And .... SCORE! The team and parents erupted! As we prepared for the other team's response, I was shouting from the side-lines that we had to stay focused and maintain our defenses because Coach Jack's team were going to hammer us hard. The kids were absolutely amazing, fending off their offense, clearing the ball way out of bounds (to burn the clock) and eventually making it to the final whistle and victory!

Patrick and everyone on the team were elated, jumping up and down with excitement and relief. What an incredible game for them. And their last one together as most of the kids aged out of the league when they started high school the following year.

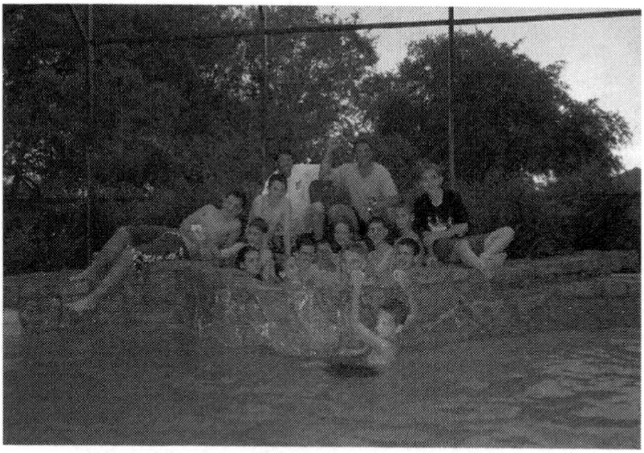

Those years and seasons playing soccer were mostly fun times for Patrick. They were hard work, with some frustration at times, but the frustration didn't last for too long. He had great memories from playing soccer and I do too. We spent a lot of father/son time together during those years and I had hoped that the lesson of struggle followed by victory would help him in the future. Perhaps it did, but for him the struggle was ultimately victorious.

Hermit Crab

I was dreaming about a *hermit crab* when I awoke this morning. I was watching it crawl along the side of the road heading towards rock formations near the beach, searching for its home. I could hear cars driving down the road, not too distant from where I was watching over the little crab. I felt like I needed to make sure that the little guy made it back to his hole in the sand safely, almost like I had a responsibility to him to be sure he was ok.

In my waking state, I was also able to step back from the scene and examine what I was doing and how I was feeling. The whole situation really didn't make sense to me. First of all, why in the world was I dreaming about a tiny *hermit crab*? And why was I emotionally invested in its well-being? I had a couple hermit crabs for a sophomore biology project in high school, so maybe I was feeling guilty about how they died (someone had sabotaged the experiment by turning their heater to maximum)? Nah, that couldn't be it.

Hermit crabs need companionship and they need space to grow in, specifically they need to be able to change from smaller shells to larger ones as they grow. Hermit crabs literally carry their homes with them in the form of the shells they retract into. They live in the sand and when younger at some point they grow gills that enable them to breathe air when they are above water. As I woke more, I realized that the *hermit crab* was a metaphor for Patrick.

> Soon after graduating from high school, Patrick and his best friend, Jake, moved into our guest house which is adjacent to our home. We had built

it a couple years earlier for family and friends to stay in when they visited us, plus it would be available for either Lydia's or my parents to live in if they chose to retire to Florida. Patrick and Jake were going to UCF in the fall semester and they both wanted to move out of their parents' home and into a place of their own. Lydia and I offered the guest house to them because it would be less expensive than them getting an apartment and we'd be more able to keep an eye open for Patrick with him next door.

That first semester was disastrous for the both of them. They didn't take college seriously and they partied way too much. Over the Christmas break, Patrick confided in us that he had failed his classes, he was addicted to marijuana and he needed our help. In a drastic move, one thing we did was have Patrick move back home. And, although I had told Jake initially that he could stay in the guest house, we ultimately decided that it was best for Patrick if he didn't. I hated reneging on my earlier commitment to him, but I had to put Patrick's well-being above Jake's situation.

In the months that followed, Patrick got better. Not well, but better. Although he had crawled back to us begging for help initially, he seemed to resent having to live with us again and we rarely saw him. Sometime later I learned that he got teased by friends who insisted that he shouldn't have moved back home, but they had no idea of the full picture of what was going on with him. For a while, it seemed that Patrick resented us, although he had come to us for help. I always felt protective of him, and I wanted him to be safe and well. But there was only so much that he was willing to let us do for him.

After failing out of UCF, Patrick went to Valencia College, which is a junior college feeder school for UCF. He started getting his life back together and had a successful first semester there. Although I was testing him for marijuana use, I'm pretty sure he wasn't totally clean yet. But his behavior was much improved over the prior semester, so he was making progress. At the end of his first semester, he approached us with the desire to change homes again. Jake and he plus a friend of theirs, Stephen, wanted to get an apartment together. Patrick wasn't working, so he needed my signature on the lease and I would have to pay his rent. I was very concerned and uneasy over the thought of him moving out so soon after his meltdown several months earlier. Before I would sign the lease, I wanted to speak with Jake and Patrick together. Specifically, I wanted to hear from them that they wouldn't screw up again and that they would look out for each other. After I got their assurances, the guys moved into the apartment.

The home they had together in that apartment was pretty good, from what we heard. As Patrick continued studies at Valencia College, things seemed to be pretty good until only a few months later when Patrick voiced frustration with living there. I was surprised to hear that the situation had turned sour so quickly. "So, what's wrong?" I inquired. The response that I got was that one of his roommates wasn't doing his share to keep the apartment clean. And Patrick was wanting to break the lease and move out because of this. The more I probed into the situation the more I realized that this was another example of Patrick's pattern of fixating on something relatively minor and then turning it into a major problem in his own mind. Eventually things settled down for a while longer, but a time came when the three of them would move again. At this time, Patrick became interested in oceanography and he was accepted to Stetson University in DeLand, Florida.

Patrick's third home away from home was a studio apartment not far from the office where I worked. It was at a half-way point between his school and our home. He was super excited to go to Stetson and he was more focused than ever on succeeding at school. He was ready to work really hard in school and he wanted to excel. However, during the year that Patrick attended Stetson, he had some extremely low times. Classes there were much harder than what he was accustomed to, and he felt he must spend every waking moment focused on studying. And he did exactly that. During his final semester there, he would come to our house to study sometimes, but most of those visits were focused on trying to help him emotionally as he was having a very difficult time with the stress from his classes. I gave him advice on how to spend his time, and not try to do everything to the 100% mark because he didn't have enough time and energy to excel at everything. It didn't help that a few students died by suicide on campus during that year, and I was increasingly nervous over Patrick's mental health situation. It reached a point where he seriously considered giving up on college and joining the military like some friends of his had done. He felt like his choice had backfired on him, and he would not succeed. But he stuck with it and mid-way through the last semester he seemed to find a rhythm that worked for him. He did well in his classes, but ultimately, he left Stetson and returned to Valencia and completed an Associate in Arts (AA) degree as a step to re-applying to UCF. His switching back to Valencia was somewhat bittersweet to me because he had done well scholastically at Stetson, but the real plus self-imposed pressure was emotionally draining for him. He argued that if he stayed at Stetson, he wasn't so sure that he could hold it together. Recalling the suicides that had happened there, I agreed with his motives.

So, Patrick changed homes again, this time to a larger one-bedroom apartment not very far from our home. During his stay there, he completed his AA at Valencia, then returned to UCF and completed his undergraduate degree. As Patrick was searching for full-time employment, he came to me with the suggestion that he return to the guest house so as to reduce expenses. His suggestion surprised me somewhat, but it was a great idea. Unfortunately, we had friends living there at the time and I argued that it wouldn't be fair to kick them out again (we had done it once before with them due to other family members moving in). A couple months later, our friends surprised us when they announced that they were moving to Missouri, so Patrick returned to living in our guest house.

There was a time when Patrick had roommates, but the majority of his adult life was spent living alone. He changed homes many times along the way, with each place meeting the needs of the moment for him. For me, I always felt an undercurrent of concern for Patrick because of him being on his own. But, he preferred it that way and he didn't want us dropping in on him unannounced.

For those people in our lives that live alone, or seem to isolate themselves, how would it feel to reach out to them to let them know that we care about them and that they're not alone? I am trying to challenge myself more to do as I say, but I find the first step to be the most difficult. I struggle to find the courage regularly to connect with others partly because I was alone in my own mind for so long.

Thanks for the reminder, little *hermit crab.*

Church

Today's inspiration comes from the fact that I woke up this morning with the song *Take Me To Church* stuck in my head. I have Matt McAndrew's cover of the song from season seven of *The Voice* in my music collection and I heard it yesterday while riding my Spyder in the morning.

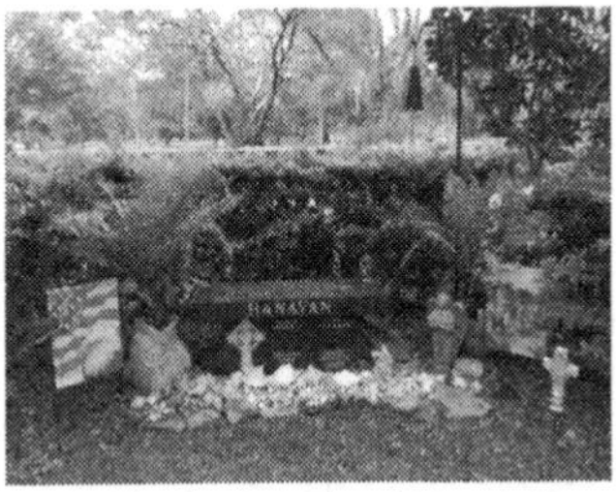

Yesterday I rode to the cemetery to visit with Patrick. While there, I cleaned up the site a bit and swapped the flags for patriotic ones as this week is July 4, Independence Day for the United States of America. Typically, I have to remove fallen branches and twigs from the site, but I didn't have to do that yesterday. After talking with Patrick for a while, I returned to my ride.

Upon departing from the cemetery, I made the decision to do something I hadn't done before – I went to where Patrick had worked although I didn't know exactly where it was located. I found it fairly easily, although there is no signage on the building. Being an e-tailer, they don't expect walk up business at all so there's really no reason for them to advertise their location. I stopped in their parking lot for a while, just soaking up the vibe of the place and thinking back to earlier times.

Like Lydia and me, Patrick was raised Catholic and we went to church regularly. Unlike some other kids, he didn't object to going to church (much) and he didn't fight against going to religious education classes. He was confirmed when he was a junior in high school and then he stopped going to church. I was very disappointed with his choice, but it was his choice to make.

When I was in college, I stopped going to church for a couple years. I worked for a clothing retailer and unlike all of the other locations, our store wasn't located in a mall and we weren't subject to the blue laws in Texas at that time. As a result, we were open seven days a week, so I also worked Sundays. I got into the habit of not going to church because my work schedule would often conflict.

Patrick didn't have the excuse I had, but he stopped going to church, nonetheless. My relationship with my son was always a bit strained, probably because I was very judgmental of him, but I never pressed him about not going to church. I didn't always agree with his choices and I rarely held back my opinions, but in this instance I respected his independence. And we hardly ever spoke about it, although occasionally I would try to nudge him to go with us.

Although Patrick didn't go to church, he was very spiritual. I recall a time when he was talking with Christine where he was sharing his thoughts on the existence of God. He communed regularly with God when he was out experiencing nature, whether doing a hike, out on his surfboard or just sitting still listening to the wind in the trees. He used a leaf to explain his view that God is at the core of the design of everything in the universe. I was amazed at how passionately he spoke about God and his feelings of being part of His creation. I took the opportunity to invite Patrick to go to Mass with us again, and he responded saying that he doesn't get the same feeling going to church. He was turned off by the structure, the repetition, the hypocrisy of some people, and he didn't like the music. Oh well, I tried.

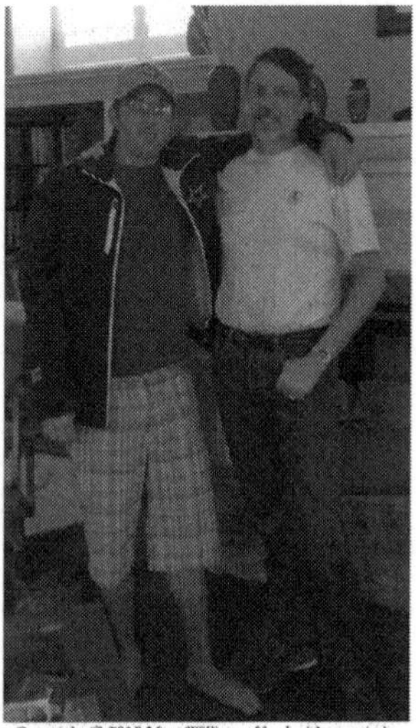

We had a funeral mass for Patrick in the same church where he was confirmed. The music was provided by friends of his and I chose the songs. Like Lydia's and my wedding, three priests celebrated the mass for Patrick - Father John (pastor), Father George, (associate pastor) and our good friend, Father Mike, who came from Augusta, GA to be with us.

Church and our faith are very important elements of my life, and although Patrick wasn't a participant in any structured religion, he believed in God. And I truly believe that he has returned home to the Kingdom of God and I know that I will see him again.

In time…

CONSEQUENCES

I have felt myself pulling away from the thought of sharing what *consequences* means to me. The word has been on my mind for a while as I have been writing but difficult memories come to mind thinking of it. Of course, there is the elephant in the room *consequence* of Patrick not getting the help he needed and ultimately taking his own life.

If this, then that.

If you do this, then that will happen.

Consequences.

It's a parental tool that we use to teach our kids about life and making the best choices. The most negative view of its use is "If you screw up and do something bad, then you will be punished." But *consequences* are also an outcome with positive reinforcement.

> I had numerous conversations with Patrick when he was younger around *consequences.* For those most significant situations or choices, *consequences* was my go-to tool. And Patrick really disliked those discussions. Even when there was a potential up-side to choices he could make, he got anxious from the stress of making decisions. So, even though I believed *consequences* to be an effective way of teaching him how to make good decisions, there was an unintended down-side from using it. The stress that often resulted wasn't something that was always obvious to me. And

for him, the added stress often meant that he felt the need for self-medication. After years of the emotional roller coaster, I felt like I was in a no-win situation. There was always the potential unexpected *consequence* from communicating *consequences* to Patrick.

After Patrick had flunked out of UCF, I was searching for something that would motivate him to get clean and stay clean. For several years I had been going to different track events and races across Florida and Georgia. I had a 1995 BMW M3 racecar (not legal for the road) that I would trailer to the track for a weekend where I would either participate in a track event with the Porsche Club of America (PCA) or I would be racing with Sports Car Club of America (SCCA). I went to the track several times a year and Patrick often went with me. In the case of PCA, he would be able to ride along with me on the track, which he thoroughly enjoyed. I made an offer to Patrick with positive reinforcement in hopes that it would help him focus on staying clean. Because my M3 racecar was expensive and a bit fragile, I offered to buy another racecar, a Mazda RX-7, that Patrick could drive on the track regularly. If he got clean and stayed clean, then we would do track weekends together with the RX-7. If he wasn't clean, I would sell the car.

Consequences

At the time, I really believed that something as significant as regular track events with the RX-7 would make a difference in his decisions. I was hoping that it was the extra nudge in the right direction for him to turn the corner and turn his life around. But, at that time I really didn't understand the full extent of his mental illness. Inadvertently, I think I actually made his life more difficult as I added pressure on him in the form of a choice he needed to make every day. I imagine that he asked himself "Do I smoke this joint so I can feel better now, or do I not so I can feel better later while racing on the track?"

I hoped that the incentive of going to the racetrack regularly would influence him to make a better decision, but I was wrong. We took the RX-7 to the track together a few times but eventually I decided to sell it because Patrick wasn't keeping up his end. When I announced my intention to sell the car, I was hoping that news might jolt Patrick into actions that would clean himself up. But by that time, he had already made his choice. At first, I wanted to be angry with him but mostly I was extremely disappointed. I felt that I failed him, and had failed as a father because it seemed that I couldn't help him. And more importantly, it seemed that he didn't want my help.

Where I had originally been so very hopeful for a positive outcome, I experienced the exact opposite

consequences.

Music

Since starting the process of writing every morning, I have rarely had a situation where I didn't find inspiration from my dream state or waking thoughts. Today was one of those days, and the theme was elusive to me at first. As you may have detected by now, I do get inspiration from songs at times and it happened again this morning.

During our drive to Georgia a week ago, we were listening to my Singles playlist. One song that played a few times, and the song that was playing in my head when I woke up today, was *Sir Duke* by *Stevie Wonder.* It speaks to music's effect on people.

> From junior high school on, music has been in my life. I never took music in school and I never learned to play an instrument, but I enjoyed listening to it. Friends from college days of mine were also into music and during the cassette-era we would share music with each other regularly. I got introduced to many recording artists from many different genres that I had never heard of before. Artists like Andreas Vollenweider, Spyrogyra, Acoustic Alchemy, Genesis, George Winston and Rush. Sadly, two of my best friends from college that influenced my tastes in music have both died, but I think about them regularly when I hear music from artists that they introduced to me.
>
> Patrick enjoyed music, too. We went to some concerts together and got to see Tool, Nine Inch Nails, Queens of the Stone Age, and Flogging

Molly. And Patrick introduced me to bands like cKy, Chevelle, Silverchair, Godsmack and Disturbed. Music was always playing from my iPod as we rode the Spyder together, so we weren't just riding with the sound of wind in our faces.

A couple years before his death, Patrick asked me for help burning some CDs. He had assembled a collection of songs that he wanted to transport without having to schlep his laptop. He didn't have a CD burner in his laptop, so he asked for my help. To make it easier for me, I copied the tracks to my iTunes collection and then burned the CDs from that. And, I recall telling him that I would keep the tracks in my collection in case he needed them burned again.

Following his death, I stopped riding the Spyder for a long while because the memories of what we had shared were very fresh in my mind and it was too painful for me to consider riding without him. Lydia was also not interested in riding, so the Spyder sat in the garage for several months. I finally stirred up the courage to get back out on it, and while updating my iPod with new music to take with me I stumbled across Patrick's playlist. I had never played it before, and I had totally forgotten that I had it. I pretty much knew that it would be painful to listen to, and I briefly considered deleting the playlist so as to avoid that pain. Instead, I copied the playlist to my iPod and went for a ride.

I waited until I was on a road near the Orlando Sanford International Airport, and I switch to the playlist. And I had to pull off the road because… well, waterworks. Tears were streaming down my face when I heard the first track which was *Always For You* by *The Album Leaf.* The song includes the lyrics

In the air I flew
Through the clouds I fall

And all the memories that were made
For years and years
I've chased this day
They were always for you
Always for you

That was enough for me to fall apart. I was only able to listen to the first couple minutes of that song and I had to stop. It seemed that Patrick was talking to me from heaven and I wasn't prepared for the onslaught of emotions that the song was stirring up in me. After a time, I switched to a different playlist and continued my ride.

Soon after, I shared that story with my executive coach at the time, Gabriela. I shared that it was hard to listen to Patrick's playlist because I found myself missing him and also thinking about what meaning those songs had for Patrick. She encouraged me to play the music, but to listen to it for myself, to see what the songs meant to me. It took a few attempts, but I did finally manage to make it through the whole playlist. The vast majority content is from artists I've never heard

> of, and much of it is rather melancholy. But for the most part, I enjoyed the music. And I felt a real connection with Patrick while riding and listening to his playlist.

Today, I still find it difficult to listen exclusively to Patrick's playlist. Rather, I hear songs from it whenever playing music randomly from my iPod. I am quick to recognize one of those songs when it starts and I listen intently to the lyrics (which is rare for me). I manage to avoid the waterworks and I try to get enjoyment from listening to a song that Patrick liked enough to make the cut for a special playlist he had assembled.

Music touches our soul and I believe we get a glimpse into the hearts of family and friends from music that they enjoy.

Alone

We don't go through life completely on our own, separated from other people. The human condition says nothing specific about other people but it's implicit in our life journey. At times, we are physically alone, all by ourselves, separated from others. And sometimes we feel alone, even when surrounded by other people.

What was your first reaction when you read the word *alone* at the top of the page? Did it stir up feelings in you? Did you identify with it because you are alone a lot? Or, did you get a sense of dread because to you *alone* has negative connotations associated with it?

> While I was younger, I often felt alone even though I grew up in a family of six. As my dad was in the U.S. Air Force for twenty years, we moved every few years and each time we moved meant starting over with school and friends. My default behavior is that I'm an introvert and I am very shy and have difficulties making friends. At any one time, I would have a couple friends at most and they weren't close friends. Other than playing soccer in junior high school, I didn't participate in many activities outside of school.
>
> I seemed incapable of breaking the cycle I was in where I journeyed through life on my own, quiet and nearly invisible to others. I had been comfortable being in my own world, isolating myself from others but I really didn't enjoy it. Then, two people came into my life and the strong feelings of being alone mostly faded away for me.

I met Edgar when I started college and he would become the best friend I ever had. He was the one who got me to come out of my shell and spend time with other people. Because of his influence on my personality, I didn't retreat into being alone when I met Lydia six months later. Three years after meeting Lydia, we got married, and Edgar was my best man.

When Patrick was young, I was so happy to see that his personality was nothing like mine had been at his age. He was very outgoing, and he had many friends. Lydia taught him how to fish, and he and friends would regularly get out in nature together. He played soccer from elementary school through middle school. Patrick had many friends and his circle of friends grew when he reached high school. He also didn't seem to suffer from the extreme shyness that I experienced, and he had a few girlfriends where I had had none.

For me, the first signs of his mental health challenges surfaced when he was in high school. At the time, I thought the issues were "girl trouble," as his girlfriend had severe mood swings from mental health issues of her own. After some turmoil from that relationship, Patrick seemed to get back to himself and everything was looking up when he graduated from high school.

After high school graduation, many of Patrick's friends moved away from Florida, and that really affected him emotionally. Some went off to college elsewhere, some to the military and others followed job opportunities in other states. He got quite down every time another one would leave. Patrick's circle of friends was huge in comparison to my experience and I even commented to him a few times that he had been very blessed to have had so many friends. One moving away didn't mean that the friendship was over, rather, it just made staying in touch more difficult.

More friends moved away. More friends got married and he would see them less and less. He did meet some new friends in college, but he never had a steady girlfriend after high school. Over the course of his years in college, Patrick became more and more *alone*. He lived alone. He surfed alone sometimes. He would go by himself on nature hikes. As his mental health struggles increased, he retreated more and more into his shell.

We were aware of changes in his life that were affecting him, and we tried our best to help him understand and cope with the changes that happen in life. But such was his state of mind that he couldn't get past the negatives. He would dwell on the negatives, over and over and over. And he felt more and more *alone*.

The fact is, we are not *alone* on our life journey. We may feel *alone* but there are others we can turn to, be it family or friends. So many times when we hear of someone's suicide it is accompanied by comments of "We didn't know." My hope is that those of us who struggle less with mental health issues can help those who are *alone* and struggling. I can tell you that it is not an easy thing to do, but I would rather help those people in my life instead of attending their funeral.

Holidays

I woke up this morning with mixed feelings because the anniversary of Patrick's death is approaching, followed two days later by Lydia's and my wedding anniversary. Thinking of the opposites of extreme sadness and extreme joy makes me recall the rollercoaster of emotions that often came around *holidays* for us.

> Holidays were often challenging for my family, mainly because we never knew what mood Patrick would be in around that time. For some unknown reason, Patrick seemed to direct his foul mood at Lydia, and she bore the brunt of his short temper and sarcasm. And the most dreaded days were around Mother's Day and Lydia's birthday. My belief is that Patrick would be difficult to be around because of frustrations with seeing others in a really good mood. It would remind him all the more that he didn't feel the same as them.
>
> But, Patrick's dark mood would seem to lift on Christmas day. And around Christmas, he really enjoyed showing us nearby homes he had found that were decorated to the extreme, like Clark Griswold did in *National Lampoon's Christmas Vacation.* One such house was in Winter Park, and we visited it multiple times each year.

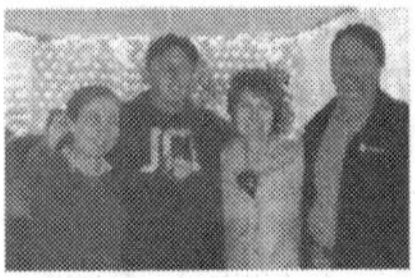 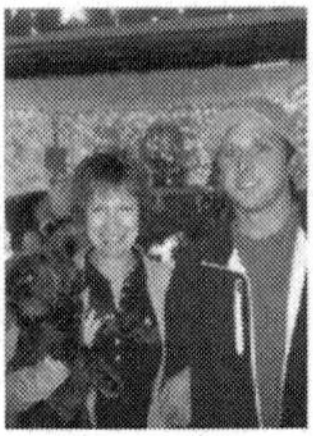 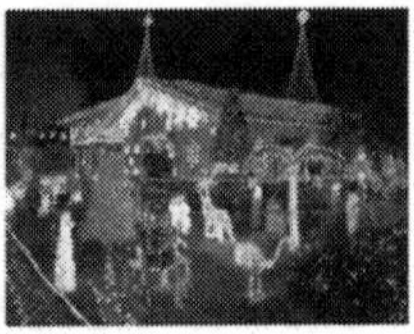

One holiday with very positive memories for me was Father's Day 2011. Patrick, Lydia and I went to lunch together at our favorite lunch spot in Winter Park, Florida. I had something in mind that I wanted to discuss with them, and I brought it up when I found the right time in our conversation. I had wanted a motorcycle for several years. Specifically, I was interested in a Harley Davidson V-rod which was their first water-cooled motorcycle. More than a decade earlier, Porsche had transitioned from air-cooled to water-cooled engines for the 911 and Harley Davidson approached Porsche to help them in the endeavor. Because of Porsche's influence on the project, I was very interested in the bike.

On my iPhone, I opened a picture of a V-rod to show Lydia and Patrick, and announced "I'm really interested in getting one of these." In a split second, Lydia's response was "No way." I felt like Ralph from *A Christmas Story* when he blurts out to his mother:

> *I want an official Red Ryder carbine action 200-short range model air rifle.*

And the immediate response from her was:

No. You'll shoot your eye out.

Thinking quickly, I decided to try another tactic. I figured that Patrick would be on my side, and he would help me convince Lydia that I should get a V-rod. I turned the phone towards him and before I could say anything, he said "Mom's right. Motorcycles are too dangerous. I know too many friends who have been seriously injured on them."

Whoa! This hadn't gone the way I had hoped, or expected. At the very least, I expected to get into a discussion of the pros and cons of the idea but the notion had been rejected outright. Hmm… It was time to regroup and try yet another tactic.

I opened a different picture on my iPhone and showed it to the both of them saying "What about this one?" Surprisingly, that question was met with "That's a possibility." I had shown them a picture of a Can-Am Spyder. A friend had gotten one during the prior year, and I was intrigued by them. I hadn't really done any serious research on them prior to trying to sell them on the motorcycle idea, and when I suggested it to Lydia and Patrick I really didn't think they would agree. What a great Father's Day gift! I had permission to at least look into the possibility.

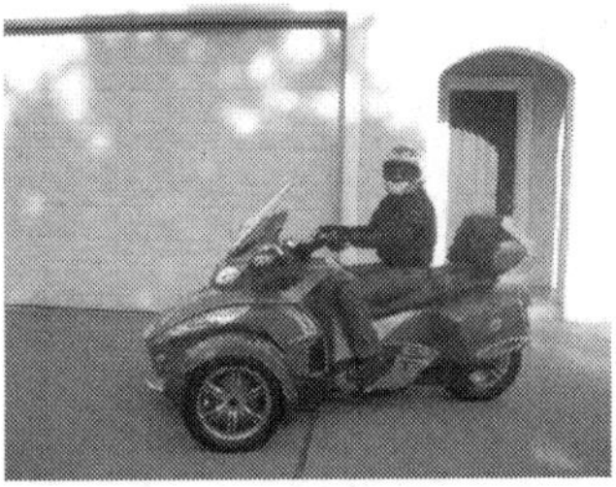

It took me a couple months to find what I wanted and I bought a pre-owned Spyder RT from a guy in Titusville. The bike sat in the garage for over a month until I could get my motorcycle endorsement on my license, and in September 2011 I took it out for my first ride. After that, Lydia and I would meet up regularly with other riders to participate in group rides and Patrick and I would go out often together. Many of my fondest memories of him are from rides we did together, especially to parks in Central Florida he introduced to me.

Today, holidays and birthdays are very different for my family. Different and difficult. We often feel the need to "hunker down" at home or in a hotel room somewhere to get through the day without Patrick being with us.

I encourage you to be especially mindful of others around the holidays. Those struggling with mental illness need us all the more at that time. The heightened emotions in others combined with the stress and expectations of holidays can drive people deeper into depression. See how they are showing up with you, and reach out to help and support them.

Beacon

Yesterday with the 4th of July, Independence Day, and for the past few years we have gotten together with neighbors to celebrate with fireworks. In addition to fireworks, last night we launched a couple of paper lanterns, one in memory of Patrick, and the other in memory of Joe, my neighbor's father who died a couple of weeks ago. The paper lanterns are like miniature hot air balloons that silently float into the sky, get caught by the prevailing winds and are carried a long way away from where they are launched. To me, the launching of the lantern was a reminder that Patrick has transcended our current plane of existence and is far away from us now. Although not with me physically now, Patrick appeared last night as a *beacon* in the sky in the form of the lantern which remained on the horizon for much longer than I expected, heading south from our house.

> A *beacon* in my life was Edgar, my best friend whom I met while I was going to college. Before I knew him, I had become very accustomed to being alone, staying at home and not experiencing life other than going to school.
>
> Curiously enough, my friendship with Edgar started on a day when I had gotten lost. I left my parents' house headed out to go to what I thought was a nearby public library. Having been in San Antonio, Texas for only a couple months, I really did not know my way around the city. And I mistakenly thought that Wurzbach Road and Harry Wurzbach Road were the same thing. I drove to where I expected to find the library, but

it was not there. I wasn't sure what was wrong, so I drove all of the way to the end of Wurzbach Road and still did not find it. After that, I wandered aimlessly around because I was certainly not going to stop and ask for directions! Eventually, I stumbled across a public library on Vance Jackson Road and I could finally start working on the research paper assignment for my English class.

When I walked into the library, Edgar was sitting at one of the tables and we recognized each other. We had met at church a few weeks earlier. Edgar was also there working on a research paper. Mine was focused on Stonehenge and he was studying seppuku (Japanese Samurai ritual suicide by self-disembowelment by sword). After a few hours of research, we were both getting ready to leave. That evening, Edgar was going with friends to the carnival at the annual San Antonio Stock Show and Rodeo and he invited me to join them. I had never done anything like that. Other than going to a few concerts when I was in high school, I had never gone out with a group of friends for dinner followed by going to an event. Although I felt a bit uneasy, I accepted Edgar's invitation. I had a great time that evening, and I was surprised at myself for having taken the step to expand my horizons.

Not only did that invitation start the process to get me out of my shell, Edgar was a *beacon* to me showing me aspects of life that I had shied away from or had ignored. We became best friends, and with other friends of his we went out for pizza and a movie on many weekends. One of my first jobs was also with Edgar, where together we managed seven newspaper delivery routes for a couple years. Remember what I said earlier?

You never know what you will find when you get lost.

A couple of decades later, I was a *beacon* for Edgar where I urged him to get a liver transplant. He had gotten infected with Hepatitis-C as a result of blood transfusions he had during surgery when he was very young. After other treatments had been exhausted, in many ways he had given up on life. He was drinking a crazy amount of beer every day and was not going to recover from it if he continued. While on a business trip to Austin, I reached out to him to see if we could get together. I drove to San Antonio and we had dinner together followed by going to see a Spurs game (Edgar was a season ticket holder, and he went to nearly every home game). My primary purpose in seeing Edgar that evening was to get him to turn his life around. He needed to get clean, admitting himself to a facility to get help, if needed. I told him that in support of his journey, I would stop drinking, too. All evening I kept telling him "You can do this" and "Your family needs you." At the end of the evening, he committed to try. That was all I needed to hear. I spoke with Edgar practically every day while he was in rehab, supporting him and giving him as much encouragement as I could. And he completed the program and got on the path to recovery.

The combination of Hepatitis-C and drinking had damaged his liver beyond recovery, however, and in early 2004, Edgar was approved for a liver transplant. He was extremely nervous about it, though, worried that he would not survive the surgery. I impressed upon him that having the transplant was his only hope of survival and he should have faith in his doctors. I wanted to be there for him when he went in for surgery, but I had just started a new job in Florida, and I convinced myself that I couldn't be there for him in person.

The transplant surgery itself was deemed a success, however, he had internal bleeding that the doctors could not stop. During a follow-up surgical procedure to stop the bleeding, a blood clot went to his brain and he had a massive stroke that he didn't recover from. I immediately flew to Texas to be with him, but it was too late. He could not talk and he didn't seem to be cognizant of what was happening to him. I put headphones on his ears and played music for him that I knew he would enjoy. And I talked with him, hoping that I could get some sign from him that he was still with me. Tears ran down his face, and it tore me up as they seemed to be saying "I told you so" to me. The nurses said it was just a reflex, and that he wasn't reacting to me but it still hurt seeing those tears. Medical science was keeping him alive via a respirator, feeding tube and pain killers. Ultimately, the decision of whether to continue this existence was with his wife, and she thankfully

> had the medical team "pull the plug" later that night. Edgar died within a few hours.
>
> I cannot tell you the number of times I have berated myself for not being there for Edgar before he went in for his surgery. For many years thereafter, I fixated on the potential butterfly effect that might have happened had I been there. I argued with myself that he would still be alive if I had been there before he went in for the transplant surgery. Although I felt that I had been a *beacon* for Edgar when he needed me, I also felt that I let him down when he needed me most.

Seeing the lantern silently float away last night, I felt several things: separation, sadness, helplessness and melancholy. But I did feel peace, too. Peace because I knew that although Patrick is not with us now, I can still see him in my memories, and I know that he is at peace. And after this morning's reflection, I now wish I had also lit a lantern for Edgar last night. Next time…

We can have a positive impact on others. We can be *beacons* to them, showing them that life's journey is worth experiencing and helping them steer away from the rocks.

Selling

Luke woke me up again pretty early this morning, partly because I didn't close the doors to the master bedroom part of our house. As a result, I experienced his favorite "Time to feed me" ritual again. I can't recall now what I was dreaming about, but the word *selling* was front and center in my mind.

Pay attention to how people talk with you and you will find that people are *selling* to you more often than you realize. This has become a bit of a joke where I work as our CEO uses *selling* as a tool in his interactions with others. A by-product of the onsite/offsite I mentioned in the introduction is that we now have the permission to call him out when we think he's transitioned into *selling* used cars to us.

Whether you are aware of it, or not, we are all constantly *selling* even if we don't have a job in Sales. And we do it with family, friends, co-workers, customers, or basically anyone we interact with.

> A few nights ago, Lydia and I were at our favorite Mexican restaurant which is undergoing a rebranding over the next few months. The owner has multiple locations that were initially launched as different brands, although the menus were mostly the same. In a move to consolidate and simplify operations, they chose to re-brand all of their restaurants under a single name and reduce to a single menu. It made perfect sense to me, as it's a move to reduce costs and increase profits for the business. They are transitioning to the new

brand in phases and we saw the new menu for the first time Friday evening. As we were finishing dinner, a couple sat down next to us at the bar, and they proceeded to complain about the changes with the head bartender, whom we consider a friend. But that wasn't enough for them, as they went on to try to convince us (i.e., *sell* us) that the restaurant owners were making huge mistakes that would cost them business. After attempting to *sell* them on why it made sense for the business, I got frustrated and said something along the lines of "Feel free to stop eating here as it will make it easier for us to get seats at the bar." And I walked away. I was tired of the useless debate as it was clear that neither of us were going to *sell* the other on their way of thinking.

Patrick had a couple of commission based part-time jobs in sales earlier in his college career. Frankly, he struggled with those jobs as he felt that he was required to be dishonest with people at times. He didn't make a lot of money doing it, but he did gain some good experience working and dealing with people.

He got a job with an e-tailer after graduating with his business degree, and their entire business was focused on *selling* goods online. Patrick started in the warehouse where he would pull inventory for orders and pack it for shipping to the customer. After a time, he moved into a combo-role of customer service and marketing. On the marketing front, he worked on the re-brand of the business and came up with their new company name (for which he received a bonus). Previously, they had operated under four different brands.

From his experience in customer service, Patrick found that the company was wasting money from their shipping choices. He took the initiative, on his own time, and did extensive research to prove his hypothesis. At this period of time, he was super engaged and really excited about the work he was doing because he believed he could make a big impact on the profitability of the business. He shared his research with me when he believed he had proof that would show that the company was overpaying on unnecessary priority shipping. He was a bit concerned, however, because he wasn't sure how to pursue the matter. I encouraged him to show his findings and recommendations to his manager, and that person would decide on whether to take it to the owner. Patrick then *sold* his views, data and recommendations to management, and the company made changes that would save the business tens of thousands of dollars every year without compromising customer service.

I was really proud of my son, and I told him so. I was proud that he took the initiative and proud that was able to sell management on making key changes that would improve the company's profitability. I thought things were going great for Patrick, and that he had progressed to the point where he had turned a corner in his mental health battle. But that view didn't last very long as a couple weeks later I detected another serious low point for him. I asked Patrick what was bothering him…

> "Remember that shipping project I worked on, where I did all of this work on my own time and got the company to make changes?"
>
> "Yes, and you did an awesome job with that."
>
> "The owner believes that it was my manager's idea and I just contributed a little. I thought I would get more recognition for what I did, and maybe a bonus."
>
> After a brief silence, I followed up saying "It's perfectly fine for you to approach the owner and clarify your involvement in the project. After all, it wouldn't have happened if you didn't take the initiative to begin with."

I don't recall what transpired next but suffice it to say that what started as an extremely positive experience turned out to sour Patrick's view of the owner, manager and the company. And he would fixate on that over the months that followed. He shared his frustrations with friends of his, who in turn encouraged him to get a job elsewhere. I did as well, but by that time I had seen the same pattern many times before and I really wasn't sure what was best for him.

Without intending it, we can cause further pain for those who are struggling with mental health challenges. Think back. How often might you have said things like:

There's nothing wrong with you. It's your imagination.

You need to stop feeling sorry for yourself.

Why are you always moping around? Can't you see that there's nothing to be worried about?

Stop moping around all of the time.

If you're going to act that way, maybe you should just go home.

Why are you so depressed all of the time?

That shouldn't have upset you.

For someone having a hard time with life's challenges, hearing these types of questions or comments does not help their current situation. Instead of trying to *sell* those people on our view of the world, perhaps we can start a different conversation that starts with

"You seem to be hurting now. Can I help you?"

Please be aware that many people will initially respond with "I'm okay" or "I'm fine." But I urge you to trust your gut and probe further. Let the other person know that you care about them, and you are inviting them to share their burden with you.

Recognizing how people are showing up, and then inviting them to be open with you could be the first step to start their healing.

PICK UP THE PIECES

I awoke this morning with a few lines from Joe Bonamassa's song *Pick Up the Pieces* playing in my head:

> *But I pick up the pieces*
> *Pick up the pieces and go*

Funny thing is, I also recalled listening to the song *Pick Up the Pieces* by Average White Band while riding the Spyder yesterday morning. Same title, but totally different song than Joe's. Those few words are a good summary of the mode I went into after Patrick's death.

> Patrick's life had been snuffed out, and I felt that mine that been shattered into pieces. The gut wrenching soul searching that came from losing Patrick was immense, and at the same time I was extremely concerned for Lydia and Christine. I felt numb and not in control of what I was doing during the days leading up to the funeral.

> I knew I had responsibilities for planning Patrick's funeral, but there was an emotional train wreck going on within me. But, I HAD to keep it together. I got strength and support from my father, who had dealt with planning many funerals. I asked him to help me out, advise me and most especially to keep an eye out for anyone trying to take advantage of us. And he helped me a lot, which I really appreciated.

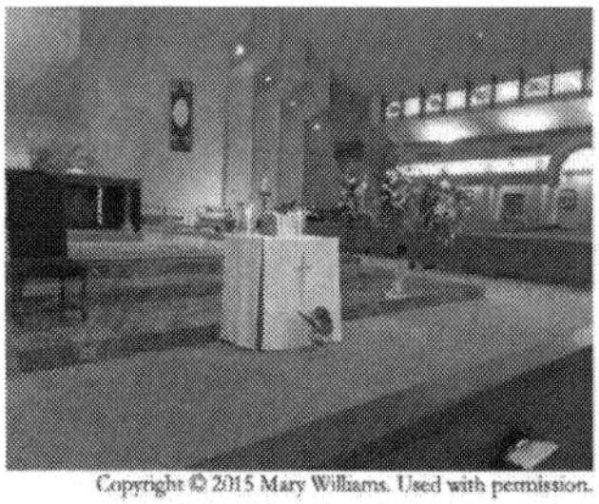

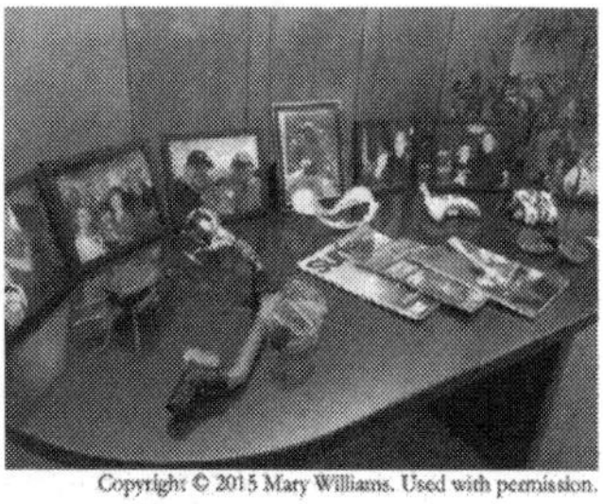

Family were quick to respond, and parents and siblings from Texas, Georgia and North Carolina came to provide their love, support and comfort to us. They were here to help us in any way possible to *pick up the pieces* and go on. So many people provided food to us over the following weeks, and I am ashamed that we could not find the strength to send thank you notes to everyone.

I recall telling people that death is part of life, and life goes on. Knowing that intellectually didn't guarantee that I absorbed it emotionally, however. The weeks, months and years that have followed still represent aspects of *pick up the pieces.*

Occasionally, I still have instances where I detect that a piece has fallen to the floor again. And I need to pause, take a deep breath, compose myself and pick up the fallen piece.

Today will very likely bring back memories of Patrick's funeral, as we will be attending the funeral of a neighbor's father who passed away last month. I expect it to be even more poignant because it will be in the same church, with the same priests and with the same cantor and pianist.

Since I am already looking backward, I'd like to take this opportunity to share the eulogy that I did for Patrick's funeral. When I was writing this eulogy a few years ago, I felt compelled to include a plea for people to pay attention to others as well as themselves. If I'm recalling correctly, Christine brought that idea into focus for me, suggesting that I use the opportunity to bring mental illness into the light so as to start breaking down the stigma. This was the seed planted in me that has grown into this book years later.

Memories of Patrick

St. Stephen Catholic Community
August 13, 2015 2:00 PM

First of all, on behalf of the Fitzgibbons and Hanavan families we want to thank you all for coming together with us to celebrate Patrick's life. It means everything to us that he was loved by so many and that you've come here from around the country to remember him.

Patrick seemed most at peace when outdoors, either hiking, enjoying the beach, fishing, surfing or Spyder riding with me. He saw God and creation in nature, and he felt more at peace in those settings. In recent months, Patrick took Lydia and I to many new parks and sites that we had never seen before. He took great joy in sharing God's creation with us.

He loved the outdoors and learned to fish when he was in elementary school. He was an amazing fisherman, and he taught many of us how to fish. A friend of his recently told us that "Patrick could pull a 7-pound bass out of a puddle." He was very serious about fishing and would use Google Earth to find new potential fishing holes and would then go to those places after school or work to check them out and see if they were worth visiting regularly. In addition to the closeness to nature that he would experience, fishing helped Patrick distance himself from his pains and struggles.

Early mornings, Patrick would go out on "dawn patrol" surfing with many of his friends. He got really excited when hurricanes were in the area. He and friends would head out to the beach in hopes of catching bigger waves than what are usually seen here. I was always nervous when they did this, but the gleam in my son's eyes was such that I just wished them "Good luck and stay safe."

After I got a Can-Am Spyder motorcycle a few years ago, Patrick would go out riding with me regularly. Again, he used Google Earth to look for new and interesting roads, routes and places to visit. Spyder rider friends of ours have enjoyed the fruits of those explorations that Patrick and I did together. He was always hunting for new roads and new places to explore, and he was so pleased to show us something new that he had found.

Even from a young age, Patrick struggled with depression so although we are shocked to our very core at losing him, the sad fact is that we are not surprised that he could not continue. He was very private, and although he had an infectious smile and seemed to be happy to most people, deep inside he was hurting and struggling with many aspects of living. I imagine that the vast majority of you had no idea about his struggle; he hid it very well. I mention this because so many people suffer in silence and alone.

If you've been asking yourself, "Why?" or "What did I miss?" or "Why didn't he come to me?," please know that it wasn't for any lack on your part and it wasn't your responsibility in any way. He didn't want you to hurt with him. What we could and did do was help him to fight as long as he could.

Depression can affect anyone – your children, your spouse, your friend, your co-worker. If you've struggled or are struggling with mental illness yourself, please reach out to your loved ones to get their love and support, and find things that help you cope. There are so many resources available to help you. Help your loved ones with mental illnesses by supporting them with your unconditional love. Never judge them for being sick and remember to take care of yourself, too.

Christine has something she wants to share with all of you:

> As I lay awake Monday morning, I pressed so close to my half-awake Dad that he got a little annoyed because I was very warm and he told me to give him some space. So I laid down flat between my parents. After a little while, I felt a strong hand hold my upper arm and I felt Patrick right there over me. He looked so happy and so healthy. There was no more pain or weariness in his eyes. His smile was big and beautiful. He looked very tan, and a little bit pink, because no matter how many times Mom pleaded with him to wear sunscreen, he never really took that

> to heart. When he spoke, he was so relaxed. The last few weeks, he had been drifting away and was so tired. But not when he came to me. All he said was, "Come on, sis," like it was so obvious that I needed to stop hurting so deeply and know that he was finally at peace. He is in Heaven and God is so good.
>
> At first though I was so confused and sat up and asked my dad, "Am I crazy? Did you feel that?" Dad was half-awake, though, so he didn't really get what I was asking. I grabbed Mom and Dad's hands and I made them sit up with me so I could tell them what had just happened. We prayed together and thanked God and Jesus, and Patrick for giving us that gift of coming to me. I couldn't stop weeping and laughing and giving praise. After I'd spent a while journaling about that gift, I heard Patrick tell me to go to sleep now. I felt his big strong arms hold me and I finally rested. Thank you so much, Patrick. Thanks be to God for giving us that blessing.

In closing, let me say that we are comforted by God's love for us and by the knowledge and conviction that Patrick is no longer in pain. Patrick is surfing with Jesus. It's dawn. They don't need any boards, and it's a perfect wave every time.

Sadly, Patrick gave up on life. The journey had become too difficult for him, and he decided it was time for him to rest. But it isn't time for the rest for us. Rather, it's time for us to reach out and help those that need us so that we're not left to *pick up the pieces.*

“Best Day of My Life”

How would it feel to hear those words from a loved one or a friend after you had spent time with them? It isn’t something you aspire to, necessarily. But if and when it happens, it must feel pretty amazing.

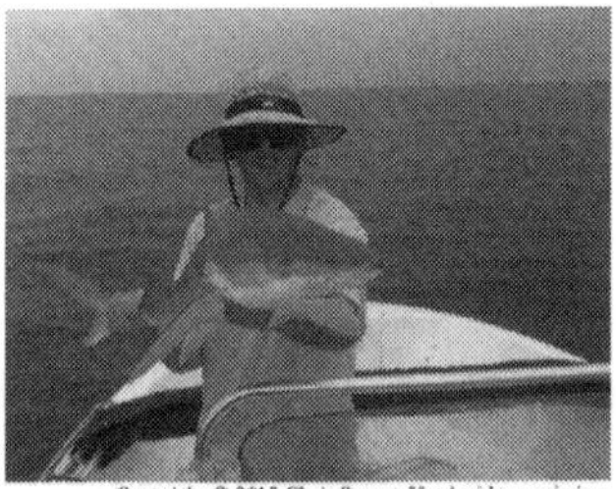
Copyright © 2015 Chris Bower. Used with permission.

Patrick made the pronouncement of *"best day of my life"* following a fishing trip he did with friends on July 4, 2015. They had gone out shark fishing in the Atlantic Ocean and they caught a lot of fish and had a great time together. Because of the remote location they went to in the ocean, he shared the GPS co-ordinates with me because he had plans to go back there again.

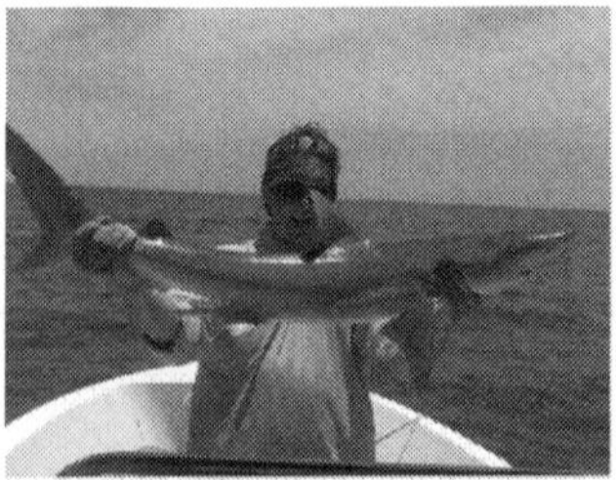
Copyright © 2015 Chris Bower. Used with permission.

Sure enough, the earlier shark fishing expedition had been so successful, that they decided to repeat it a week later. Once again, Patrick returned home excited about the good times they had while fishing that day.

Patrick seemed to be having a great summer, you might say the *best of his life*. Issues at work seemed to have quieted down and he was exploring new fishing spots in the ocean with his buddies.

For the last weekend of July and first weekend of August 2015, Patrick spent a great deal of time with Lydia and me. That was quite unusual, as he usually had "better things" to do with his time than spend it with us. It wasn't unusual for us to make plans that included Patrick, but then have him cancel out at the last minute because something better had come along, be it fishing, surfing, or some other activity with friends of his. It could be frustrating for us at times, but it was a deal we had made with him many years earlier. As our focus was on his mental health, we willingly stepped aside for him to do something that he would enjoy more. So, it was unexpected for him to want to be with us so much.

On those weekends in the summer of 2015, Patrick came to our house and asked if we had been to some places on the Florida east coast. To me, it was a continuation of how we tested each other regarding new roads we hadn't ridden yet and I was intrigued. He suggested we go to these places, and have lunch together while in the area. You could have knocked me over with a feather because this was so out of character for him. We readily agreed, and off we went.

On Saturday, July 25, 2015, as part of celebrating Lydia's birthday Patrick joined us for the day. We first went to The Breakers for lunch, a restaurant Patrick had not been to before. Then he took us to see Smyrna Dunes Park which is the northern most point of the peninsula of New Smyrna Beach. There is a nice boardwalk there, and we walked through the park on the way to the beach. I took this selfie with the three of us on our way back to the car.

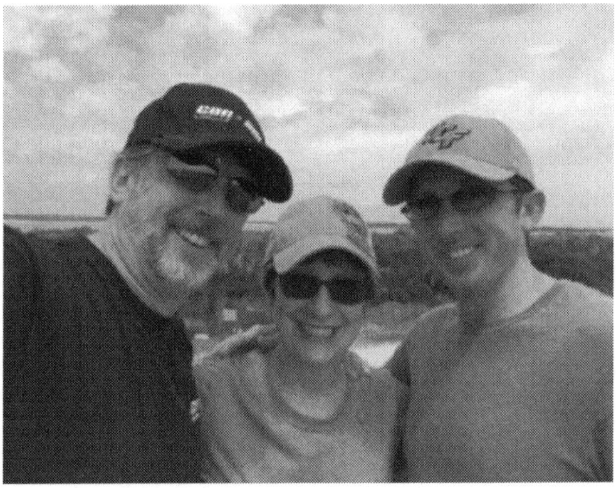

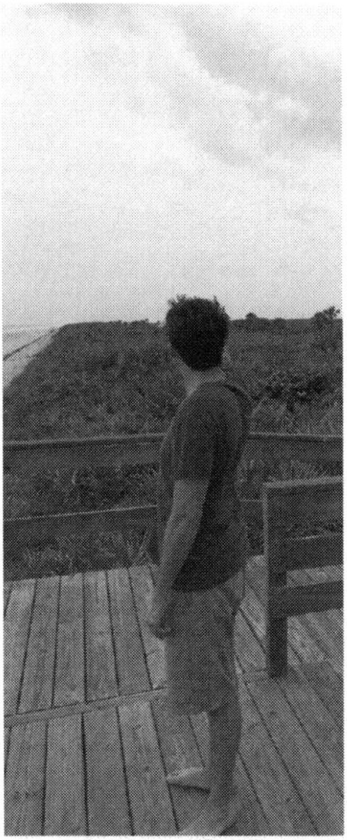
Last picture of Patrick

And on the following Saturday, August 1, 2015, Patrick surprised us again when he suggested we go to Canaveral National Seashore, which is south of New Smyrna Beach. We went to Chases on the Beach for lunch and then headed south to the park. We stopped at Turtle Mound and Playalinda Beach (but not the nude area). We had a great day together, enjoying nature, being at the beach, hearing the waves crash on the shore and feeling the wind in our faces. I spoiled the mood a bit because I was worried about the potential for rain, but Lydia and Patrick were enjoying the beach so much that they ignored my suggestions to get back to the car. It did rain on us as we headed back to the car, but that hardly mattered because we had had such a great time together.

Those two Saturdays in the summer of 2015 rank high on the *best days of my life.*

Looking back now, I can see a pattern of Patrick's actions and behaviors that were leading up to his suicide. Yes, we had some wonderful times with him that summer, but I'm pretty sure now that he was doing that to give us new memories of him before he left us.

When I took that last picture of him, I wasn't sure what he was doing at first. He was very intent looking down the beach, and he seemed to be almost absorbing the scene with his eyes. Now, I believe he was committing the view to memory to take it with him on his next journey. This area of Florida, Canaveral National Seashore, was his favorite place and he shared it with us before he left us. I am thankful that he spent the time with us that day and I'd like to believe that it was one of the *best days of his life.*

Thinking about loved ones or friends who are struggling, how would it feel to give them a *best day*? Maybe it would take some planning, but it doesn't take much to make an impact. Spending quality time with someone, perhaps enjoying nature together, taking a walk together while catching up with them on their life journey or enjoying a nice meal together can all make a difference in someone's life. Give it a shot.

RADIOACTIVE

Waking up each morning with the intent of finding that word or phrase that inspires me to write feels a bit like the old television game show *Password.* When the password was handed on a card by the host to the contestants, the announcer quietly told the audience "The password is ____." Well, today's password, or inspiration, is *radioactive* and it's on my mind for the simple reason that I awoke with the song from Imagine Dragons stuck in my mind. A few lines from that song are:

> *I'm waking up to ash and dust*
>
> *I'm waking up, I feel it in my bones*
> *Enough to make my systems blow*
> *Welcome to the new age, to the new age*
> *Welcome to the new age, to the new age*
> *Whoa, oh, oh, oh, oh, whoa, oh, oh, oh, I'm radioactive, radioactive*
> *Whoa, oh, oh, oh, oh, whoa, oh, oh, oh, I'm radioactive, radioactive*

The most common definition of *radioactive* concerns nuclear radiation that results from exploding atomic bombs. On the surface the song's lyric seems to use this definition, but the author was using it as a metaphor for becoming self-empowered. Dan Reynolds has said publicly that he was coming out of a difficult time and had suffered with depression for many years. And he changed his outlook on his own life by embracing who he was.

> In many respects, I felt that I was walking on eggshells around Patrick most of the time, afraid that he might explode. At any one time, I really

didn't know how he was feeling or what state of mind he was in then. I was concerned about upsetting him by saying the wrong thing. Sometimes I would inadvertently trigger him, but there were also some times where conversation got more heated between us and I didn't care if I upset him. The worst example of this happened when Patrick was in high school.

From what I recall, it happened during the time that Patrick was dating "blondie," who I mentioned in the *Escape* chapter. I overheard Lydia and him arguing about something in his room. I don't really recall the details, but it got pretty loud and I got upset with how Patrick was shouting at his mother. I went upstairs with the intent of diffusing the argument, but instead I got involved in it. At some point Patrick directed an f-bomb at us and I snapped. I was so upset with him for how he was treating his mother that the frustration and anger in me exploded and I slapped Patrick in the face. I immediately regretted it, and I tried to apologize, but the damage had been done. I had never done that before, and I was extremely worried that I had permanently damaged my relationship with my son. Lydia was also extremely upset with me, and she came to Patrick's defense. Instead of Patrick having been the cause of the turmoil of the moment, the blame shifted completely to me.

Sometime later, Lydia told me that our relationship had been severely damaged by my action and it was going to take a while for her to move beyond it. When she told me that, I felt like I had been punched in the gut. It was absolutely essential for me to repair the relationship with Patrick, and I went about doing what I could to mend the hurt. I sat down with him and apologized profusely and assured him that I would never do it again. He listened, but seemed to not believe me and he didn't respond to my plea for forgiveness. Perhaps he left me in limbo on purpose so that I would continue to feel pain from my actions. A few days later I checked with him again, and he acquiesced and forgave me.

That split second when I chose to slap Patrick in the face stands out to me as one of the worst decisions I ever made in my relationship with my son. But another haunts me, too.

During the year leading up to Patrick's suicide, he was constantly dealing with a roller coaster of emotions at work. He reached a point where he wanted to quit his job and he came to talk to me about it. As someone who has recruited for and hired a lot of people, I was concerned about the optics on his resumé if he had a gap in employment. A prospective new employer would see the gap and might not even consider him because it would look like he had been fired from his prior job. I encouraged Patrick to seek out a new job while continuing his current job and I offered to help him polish up his resumé and help him with practice interviewing. I told him to work his network, reaching out to friends to see if they knew of job openings that might interest him. All

> of my advice seemed to fall on deaf ears, however, as he did none of it.
>
> I am tormented thinking that Patrick might still be with us if I hadn't been so forceful with him about not quitting the job that he had grown to hate. It's another example of *woulda*, *coulda*, *shoulda* that remains very painful to recall.

Are we good at recognizing potentially explosive situations? And if so, what can we do to diffuse them? Are we contributing to triggering others and making them explode? We should try to anticipate a potential explosion, and communicate in a way so as to diffuse the situation and end with a better outcome.

Accelerate

My mind was clearly focused on *accelerate* when I was waking up, to the point where I imagined the start of writing this chapter. And then, I slammed on the brakes. I hit a wall and felt compelled to step away to collect my thoughts again.

> Over the past couple weeks, I shared a draft of this book with a few family members and close friends, and received positive feedback from everyone. My primary objective in sharing it with them was to get the answer to my question, "Would this book help people who have loved ones or friends who have mental health issues?" Everyone has responded back in the affirmative, and that has given me encouragement to continue.
>
> And then, I hit the brakes. I stopped because although Lydia said that she liked the book and believed that it would help people, she went on to say "What would Patrick think?"
>
> > Is it fair to Patrick and his memory to expose him to the world in this manner?
>
> I have mentioned earlier how private he was, and how he hid his pain from almost everyone. He isn't in pain any longer but if Patrick were still on his life's journey, and was doing better in his mental health battle, I would not be writing this book. I say that in part because mental health challenges are a constant battle. People don't get "healed," and the battle is a daily one. No doubt

> that I would make Patrick feel much worse if he were still alive and I published his story for others to experience.

I would like to believe that Patrick would want his story shared so that others might do better on their journey. But, I am really torn right now. Lydia's question "What would Patrick think?" has really made me pause and reflect.

Do I put my foot back on the *accelerator*, or do I put it in park and stop here?

Eye on the Goal

I missed a day of writing, and I am feeling the need to seek inspiration from Patrick. I opened up the text messages from him that I still have saved on my iPhone and I started scrolling back through time, recalling what was happening at those times. On the afternoon the day before my birthday in 2015, Patrick suggested a Spyder ride and had a route suggestion:

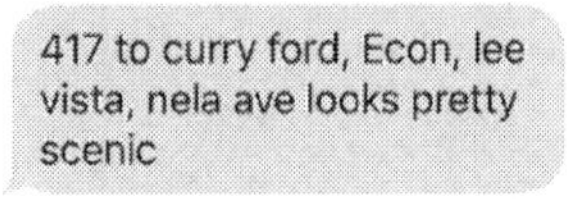
417 to curry ford, Econ, lee vista, nela ave looks pretty scenic

That route looks like this on the map:

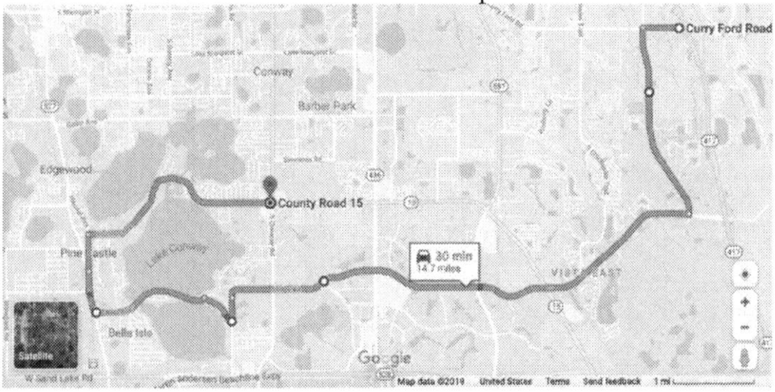

I do not recall where we rode that afternoon, but we didn't take that route, possibly because 417 is part of the local tollway system and I prefer riding on country roads with the Spyder. Having said that, it's time for some *wind therapy* this morning and I am going to ride that route now.

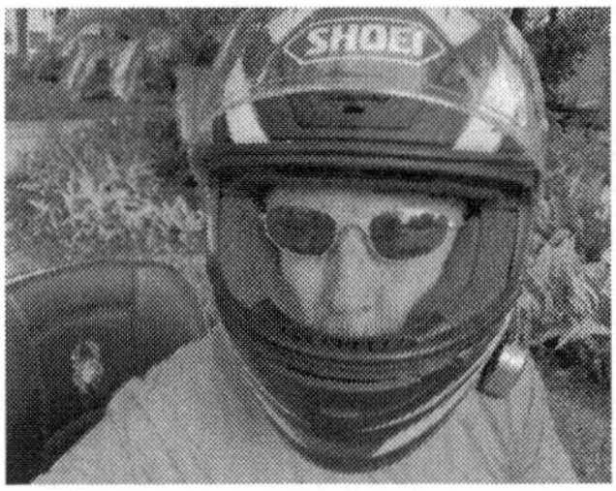

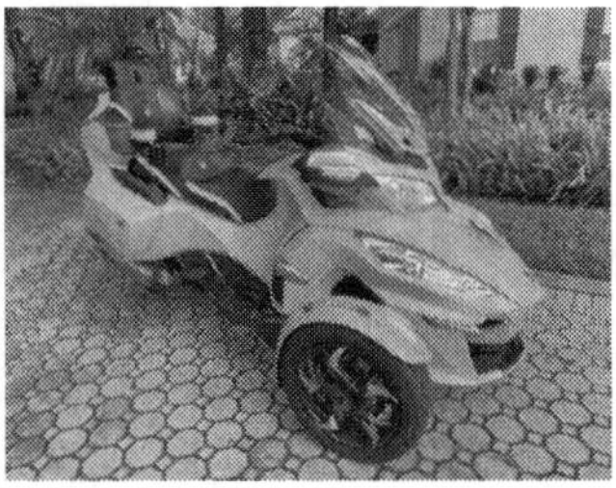

I'm back from this morning's ride and happy to report that Patrick was correct about that route being pretty scenic. He and I had ridden on Curry Ford Road, Econlockhatchee Trail and Lee Vista Blvd before but we never rode on Nela Ave and the roads around Lake Conway. It was interesting to *get lost* again, this time following a recommendation from him from a few years ago. Patrick's playlist accompanied me as I rode and I opened my heart for any signs from him about whether I should continue sharing his story.

Midway through my ride and after riding around Lake Conway, I headed south and stopped for a while at Southport Park, west of Orlando International Airport. There's an open field on the south side of the park where people regularly fly remote control airplanes on weekends. Several people were out this morning, and I stopped for a while to watch them. I recalled that I woke up this morning with the phrase *eye on the goal* on my mind. What did that mean? Was Patrick trying to respond to my unspoken question? As I was watching model planes in the sky, I took a deep

> breath, exhaled and closed my eyes. I was trying to open myself to hearing Patrick if he chose to speak to me at that moment. Thoughts of "Should I continue writing?" and "Should I publish the book?" were top of my mind. But I didn't hear anything other than the sound of the Spyder beneath me. After perhaps 30 seconds, and with a bit of disappointment, I took another deep breath, opened my eyes and shifted into reverse. And then I saw two butterflies go past the front of the Spyder. Tears immediately welled up in my eyes. Since Patrick's death, we have had numerous occasions where a butterfly would appear when we're thinking about him. To me, seeing butterflies at that moment was the answer from Patrick that I was seeking. I looked up to the sky, pointed upward and said "Thank you, Patrick."

While continuing this morning's ride, once again I considered my reasons for writing this book. My motivation remains unchanged, and given the feedback I have received thus far I feel more compelled to complete what I've started. And I don't want to repeat what I had done with Edgar when he needed me, where I decided to not fly out to see him before his surgery.

I am keeping my *eye on the goal* to help people and hopefully save lives. My hope is that sharing Patrick's story will inspire others to view mental health illness in a different light and to treat those affected differently.

Denial

Admittedly, I didn't wake up this morning with the word *denial* top of mind. I felt more like a blank slate when I woke up. Luke was doing his usual morning yowl combined with pawing at the bottom of the door to our bedroom. That caused a knocking type of sound, and it went on for a few minutes before I reluctantly got out of bed. During my short walk to the door, my alarm went off, so I couldn't be too upset with Luke for waking me early.

As I was going about the morning ritual of feeding the cats and getting Leia to do her "numbers" outside, I took mental stock of my writing progress and the topics I had hoped to cover. *Denial* immediately came to my mind, and then I started playing the song *Pretty Fly (For a White Guy)* by The Offspring in my mind. The first verse is:

> *You know it's kind of hard*
> *Just to get along today*
> *Our subject isn't cool*
> *But he fakes it anyway*
> *He may not have a clue*
> *And he may not have style*
> *But everything he lacks*
> *Well he makes up in denial*

Other than the first couple lines, the song does not remind me much of Patrick. The character in the song is someone who is pretty clueless, and Patrick was not like that. Sitting here now, it occurred to me that he might have been able to deal with life better if he had been in *denial* about those things that tormented him. His own imagination and his tendency to conclude extreme interpretations of situations caused severe mental anguish for him.

We have heard much more about depression and mental health illness in the news over recent years, either from high profile suicides or from mass shootings caused by people with mental illness. Rewind at least a couple decades and the subject wasn't discussed as much as it is today. The subject was almost taboo, and as a society we were collectively in *denial.* War veterans who returned home with severe depression were often referred to as having "shell shock," whereas today we have learned more about their plight and Post-Traumatic Stress Disorder (PTSD) is talked about more openly.

Even with there being more of a conversation and awareness around mental health, a stigma around it remains and many of those afflicted by it are afraid to speak up and afraid to get help. If we challenge ourselves to truly help those in need, we must first recognize them. Pay particular attention to how people are showing up around you. We need to open our eyes to see those who need us. Failing to see them might mean that we are in *denial.*

> I was in *denial* for many years about Patrick's mental health. When a situation happened with him, I rationalized to myself that it was just an example of adolescence, part of growing up, his imagination, or nothing serious. I had all of these escape routes I used in my own mind that avoided the cold hard fact that my son suffered from depression, or worse. I was clearly in *denial* for a very long time.

> Eventually, I woke up to the fact that he needed help and he did go to a psychologist and later a psychiatrist. In the case of the psychiatrist, Patrick had a bad reaction to some medications at first but then was prescribed something different that helped him for a while. He stopped taking the medication, however, because 1) he was feeling better, 2) he had to see the psychiatrist regularly to get refills, 3) the cost and 4) having to take time away from work. In the latter case, Patrick was so consumed with thoughts about how others would view him that he would not get help. He didn't want to have to respond to questions of "Where are you going?" or "Why weren't you at work yesterday afternoon?"

The stigma around depression and mental health survived my son. Sadly, the stigma is alive and well and he is not. If we continue to be in *denial*, we will continue losing loved ones and friends.

Stop denying what we see with our own eyes. Stop denying what we hear with our own ears. People in pain will often drop hints to us, perhaps subconsciously hoping that we will pick up on them and act upon them. They are crying out for help. We need to open our minds and our hearts to truly listen for their pleas. And, don't fall prey to the stigma, where we turn away in *denial*. If we are open and don't deny what we see and hear:

Be receptive if they reach out to you.

Acknowledge their pain.

Help heal their pain.

Talk with them.

Comfort them.

Hold them.

Love them.

Steer

Sometimes we want to get into the driver's seat of someone else's life in order to *steer* them away from a potential accident or a bad area of town. But hardly anyone is willing to let someone else take that much control of their life and *steer* them.

I don't have much time to write this morning, as I have an early morning dentist appointment. But I do have a few significant memories about Patrick that concern *steering*:

> While dating "blondie" in high school, I tried *steering* Patrick away from her by repeatedly suggesting he break up with her. She would manipulate him by threatening to break up with him if he didn't do what she wanted. I urged him more than once to recognize what she was doing to him. While dating her, Patrick experienced severe mood swings and I tried multiple times to *steer* him away from her. His mind understood what I was saying, but his heart ignored the reality that he was in pain because of her. The situation reached a point where it was clear that I had to let go of the wheel of Patrick's life and let him run off into a ditch so that he would open his own eyes and heart to fully understand how destructive "blondie" was being to him. Eventually, they did break up and Patrick's severe mood swings calmed down for a while.
>
> At times, I wanted desperately to *steer* Patrick because I was concerned about the destination he seemed to be heading towards. The most

significant of these was before Patrick started college when I sat down with him and provided advice on how to approach his classes, study habits and staying away from partying. In effect, I gave him a list of do's and don'ts so as to *steer* him down a similar path that I had taken to completing my degree. In that first semester, Patrick seemed to resist my attempts to *steer* him, however, and he mostly followed the list of don'ts. At the time, I had no idea that his mental illness had taken hold of him and that he turned to marijuana as his choice of self-medicating in an attempt to feel better. Or at least, feel numb.

During the year that we had the Mazda RX-7, Patrick had opportunities to drive it on the race track. In racing, there is an optimum "racing line" around the track which is the place where you want to *steer* the car in order to carry the maximum speed and therefore get the fastest lap time. I had many years of experience with racing and track events, and I had logged many hours and many laps on the track where we took the RX-7. I was an instructor for the Porsche Club of America, but I recommended another instructor ride with Patrick for fear that he wouldn't listen to my recommendations. Over the course of a couple weekends, Patrick got experience and did well enough that he was signed off to drive solo. And

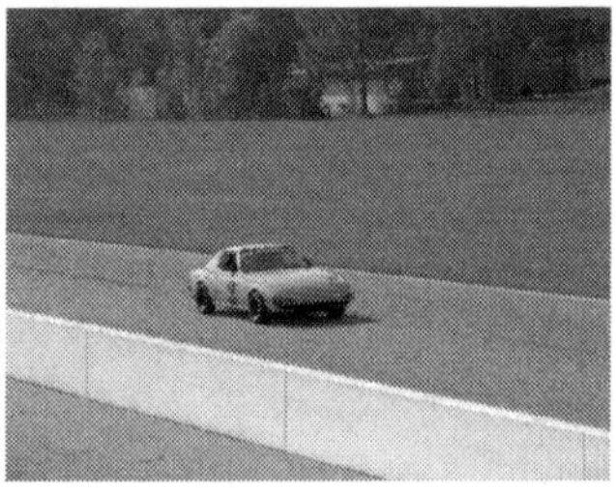

he had an awesome time on the track as he pushed the car to the limit, trying to go faster and faster.

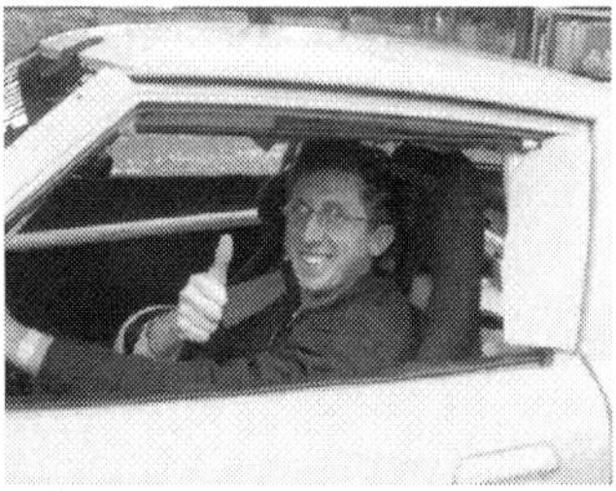

After returning home from that last weekend, Patrick worked for hours studying the video that was captured from within the car. He assembled a video and I shared RX7 Racing Montage via my YouTube channel. I was amazed at how fast his hands were on the *steering* wheel. He never lost control of the car, and he was often on the edge or a bit beyond before he *steered* through oversteer in the corner. His fast reaction times and quick hands were incredible, and I was looking forward to his getting better and better with each track weekend. It was doubly disappointing that he didn't follow through with his commitment to stay clean, and as I shared in *CONSEQUENCES*, I ended up selling the RX-7.

I had the best intentions when I tried to *steer* Patrick away from "blondie." And the same is true for wanting him to do well in college. I have a tendency to want to *steer*, where I take control of a given situation so as to achieve the desired goal. Being that controlling can be a major turnoff to other people, however, and I have to constantly resist the urge to do it.

There's a line one could cross where we stop being helpful and end up being controlling. I don't know many, if any, people who want to go through life being controlled by someone else.

Perhaps there is a better approach …

Salamander

Believe it or not, the word that was top of mind for me when I awoke this morning was *salamander.* Why in the world was I thinking about that? Then I recalled the significance for me at that moment. *Salamander* came directly from the dream I was having before I woke up, where I was in some type of trouble with a group of Italian mafia-types. One of the people in the dream was nicknamed *Salamander.* Other than a few flashes of images from my dream, I don't recall much else about it.

While doing the morning routine for the dog and cats, I pondered "Why *salamander*?" What could I possibly write about based on that word? Then I recalled that Patrick had had gecko lizards as pets at one point, but before he died he had a red-eyed tree frog named Ami, which is French for "friend." See how I connected those dots?

Salamander ➡ Gecko Lizards ➡ Red-eyed Tree Frog ➡ Ami ➡ Friend

I don't have anything significant to share about *salamander*, but I do have something to share with respect to Ami.

> When Patrick died, we had to deal with everything he had left behind, all of his "stuff." The vast majority of his stuff was given to friends of his, largely because we didn't have any use for much of it but also because we didn't want so many reminders of him around us. Plus, we were hoping that friends of his would get use out of his gear like fishing equipment, surf boards, etc.

We also needed to decide what to do with Ami. Perhaps one of Patrick's friends would take care of his cute frog, as we knew that we didn't want him. For one thing, taking care of a red-eyed tree frog is pretty involved. Ami's main diet staple was crickets. They had to be live so we would have to go get crickets for him every few days. Ugh… no thanks (Sorry, Patrick). So, we really weren't interested in taking Ami to our home. But, when we checked Ami's aquarium, he wasn't there. At first, I thought he was just doing an excellent job of hiding from us, but sure enough, he wasn't in his tank. And none of Patrick's friends knew what happened to Ami. To me, this was further evidence that Patrick had planned his suicide; it wasn't something he did spur of the moment. I really don't know why he took the time to deal with Ami instead of leaving him for us. It's another one of the "Why?" questions that I won't have an answer to in my lifetime. For some reason, I had a strong suspicion that Patrick took Ami to a nearby pet store that specializes in exotic pets and at one point I considered going there to see if I was right. But it wouldn't change anything to confirm my suspicions so I left Ami's whereabouts as a mystery.

Returning to *ami* meaning *friend…*

In addition to doing things together and spending time together, friends look out for each other. Sometimes friendships become so strong and so close, that friends become family to us. And we are even more inclined to look out for each other and take care of each other for friends who are like family. No one wants to see others in pain or suffering, be they family or friends.

> And if we see them in pain, don't we feel compelled to help in some way?
>
> If a friend were in a car accident, and they called you for help, perhaps to get a ride home because their car had to be towed away, would you help them?
>
> If a friend got cut badly at a party and needed stitches, would you be willing to help them by driving them to the emergency room?
>
> How about a friend who is dealing with a serious illness, like cancer? Do we distance ourselves from them, or help them?
>
> Do we help those family members or friends when they experience a death that affects them?
>
> What about a friend who is having a difficult time with their significant other? Or worse, someone who is going through a divorce?
>
> How do you feel when you are around a family member, friend or co-worker who seems to be depressed a lot?

We seem to be very willing to help people out with some things, but it is increasingly difficult to help out when someone's pain and suffering comes from emotionally difficult situations. And it seems to be even worse when we really have no idea why someone is in pain. Do we reach out to those people in an effort to help them? Or perhaps, we rationalize that it's best to give them space and not bother them.

It can be very difficult to find the emotional fortitude within ourselves that allows us to reach out and connect to someone who is in pain emotionally. Perhaps you are stronger than you think and you can help others in need. Have the courage to take the first step.

"You seem to be hurting. Can I help you?"

Elephant

No, I wasn't dreaming about elephants last night, but for some reason I do not understand, the word *elephant* was on my mind when I awoke. It seems that I have an animal theme going on over recent days!

"The *elephant* in the room" refers to an obvious topic that everyone is aware of, but one that doesn't get discussed because doing so would make people uncomfortable. I have been with other people where it's clear that another person is having difficulties. Long heavy sighs, failure to engage in the conversation, staring off at a single spot, having a long, sad face are all indicators that telegraph that something isn't quite right for the other person. Yet, the usual response to that person is to look the other way and ignore what's going on with them. Admittedly, I usually would not feel comfortable to speak to the *elephant* in the room and ask the person if something is wrong for fear that I would cause them pain. But I have done it. And recently, too.

> A few days after I started writing this book, I was at the office and our executive team were having another onsite/offsite. This time the executive team's focus was on the overall company strategy which we needed to revisit and refresh as it hadn't been touched in a few years. Our coach, Dr. Laura, was with us again to facilitate the process. On our last afternoon together, I started picking up cues from another person that something was wrong. He didn't seem to be paying attention to our conversation. He stared at a specific spot on the table for a while, and put his hands to his

forehead a few times. All of these behaviors were unusual for him. In addition, his wife was expecting a baby soon, and prior to the changes in his body english, he had been checking his mobile phone. To me, he was obviously troubled or in pain and his situation had turned into an *elephant* in the room.

Although atypical for me, I spoke up and asked him "Are you ok? Is something wrong?" I was genuinely concerned for him, and wondered if he had gotten bad news from his wife. Our executive team had been practicing openness with each other, so even though it felt uncomfortable for me to do so, I thought it was the right thing to do at that time for him. Thankfully, it turned out that he had been dealing with a bad headache for a few hours and we were able to get something for him to help with that.

While this example isn't as profound as one where someone is in emotional distress, I mention it because there are many times in our lives when we are with others, and someone in the room obviously needs help. And in the case of someone dealing with depression, it's like we become the *elephant* and they are the mouse. If you are unfamiliar with the premise that elephants are afraid of mice, check out episode 91 from season 7 from the MythBusters television show. Often times, we don't go so far as to ask them "Are you ok?" because we are afraid to hear the answer.

When Patrick was alive, I would usually only see him once or twice a week. He was close by, either living in an apartment or he was next door to us, but he wouldn't come visit us a lot. And, he didn't want us going to visit him. The majority of the times, his visits were unannounced and if he came over we would often change our plans in order to spend time with him, helping him if that was needed.

If things were going well, we might watch a Formula One race together, catch up on things going on in our lives, discuss a current work project, or pull the Spyder out.

But if things weren't going well, Patrick might want to sit with us in silence, get a backrub, talk about his troubles, or pull the Spyder out (for the *wind therapy*).

I found myself studying Patrick in the first few minutes that I would see him, trying to determine his mood from his body english and how he would talk. I wanted to know if he was having a good day or a bad one. Did he need our help today, or do we need to do things to not spoil his current mood? I was definitely the elephant most of the time, afraid to be the one to make the first move for fear that I would upset him or make him feel worse. And there were times when either Lydia or I would need to take point with him as the other was emotionally wrung out already.

Most times I find it difficult to approach others who are hurting emotionally and/or depressed. I unfortunately have a lot of experience with it, and that makes it easier for me now as compared to many years ago. Being easier doesn't mean that it is easy, however.

"Why do I find it difficult to reach out to others in pain?"

I have not really given that question much conscious thought and consideration. But now that I've asked it, I feel obligated to address the question instead of leaving it hanging out there.

For me, it isn't easy to hear about someone else's emotional or mental health difficulties. I often start feeling a bit down or depressed when I hear about someone else's troubles. Being that empathetic crutch for someone else to lean on is not easy, but I still choose to do it. In being open and listening, my hope is that the other person will feel better knowing that someone else cares enough to at least hear them out. And perhaps I can provide some perspectives or advice without going so far as trying to steer them.

CHECK-IN

WARNING: CONTAINS GRAPHIC IMAGERY

No, I'm not talking about the airline travel type of check-in. We need to check-in on each other occasionally, to see how we're doing. An early indicator of trouble on the horizon is when someone goes silent for long periods of time. In my experience, no news is usually bad news.

What I have suggested here is not intended to be a replacement for someone seeking professional help, either with a psychologist or a psychiatrist, or both. I strongly believe that mental health professionals can help us, and I encouraged Patrick on numerous occasions to do just that.

> After Patrick's death, Lydia often asked me to go with her when she met with her psychiatrist, Dr. Carol. I kept telling myself and her that I was fine. I was working hard to not fall into the *woulda, coulda, shoulda* trap. Life goes on, and I needed to *look forward, not backward.* Given what we had been through, Dr. Carol would also *check-in* with me to see how I was doing and during one session Lydia reminded me of some of my behavior for which she was concerned. Dr. Carol probed into what the cause might be, and I had to pause and reflect on what was going on inside me (something I rarely ever do). In my reflection, I found the source of my pain.
>
> > Tuesday before Patrick's death, we took a Spyder ride together in the afternoon. It was raining in the area, and I took a route

to stay dry as much as possible. There was very little talking going on and Patrick seemed alone in his own thoughts.

Wednesday evening before Patrick's death, I spoke to him again about getting professional help but he just sat in silence listening to me. After he went home, I told Lydia that I was very concerned for him and we should cancel our plans for our upcoming four day weekend in Savannah to celebrate our wedding anniversary. We needed to be home in case Patrick needed us.

Two days later, on Friday, I took the day off from work so that Lydia and I could have some "us" time while Patrick was at work. Lydia and I had a great day together. Although it was August, and it was pretty hot outside, we did a Spyder ride, ate lunch out and cooled off in the pool when we got home. Lydia heard Patrick come home from work early that afternoon. There had been the possibility that he was going to be required to work that weekend and I was hoping he had gotten the afternoon off to make up for his weekend getting ruined. That evening I had fallen asleep on the couch in our family room while watching television, which was unusual for me.

I was awakened around 10:15 PM by a co-worker of Patrick's calling my cellphone. He told me that Patrick had left work early and without telling anyone, which was extremely unusual. And he had gone silent, not responding to text messages or phone calls. Since it was so out of character for him, the folks Patrick worked with were very concerned. They pulled his employee file, found his emergency contact (me) and called. I thanked them for letting me know, and told them I would figure it out and get back to them.

I told Lydia about the phone call, and she wanted me to go next door and check up on Patrick. I wanted to believe that he was asleep and I knew he would be upset with me for intruding on his privacy. Nevertheless, I went next door and looked around. All of the lights were off, the television wasn't on and his car was in the garage. I opened the door and called out to Patrick, but didn't get an answer. I went into his bedroom, hoping to find him asleep in bed. It was pretty dark in the room and I couldn't tell if he was in bed, or not, so I reached into the bathroom and turned on the light so as to see the room better. And when I did that, I was immediately hit with the image of Patrick on the floor of the bathroom, lying in a pool of his own blood, dead from a self-inflicted gunshot wound to his forehead. His eyes were open and looking up, but there was no life in them. I immediately recalled the premonition I had had a few years prior, and I fell to the floor helpless and screaming. "No! NO! NO!!" and "Why?!" and "Oh, Patrick… why did you have to do that?" I felt like I had stepped off the edge of a cliff, with no support below me and I was falling and falling, and would do so forever. After several minutes of screaming and sobbing, I collected myself enough to call 911. The woman who took the call tried to get me to check Patrick's vitals, even though I had already told her that he was dead. I shouted at her, "HE'S DEAD! He's not moving, and he's ice cold. Nothing can be done now."

I went back home to deliver the horrible news to Lydia and Christine, and we all hugged, screamed and sobbed together as we stood on our front porch. The second phone call I made that night was to Father John. He immediately came to our house and as soon as he got out of his car he came towards us and said "Patrick is in heaven now." That was such a relief to hear, and it brought on a new flood of tears. Our very good friends, Alice and Pat, also came to be with us and they stayed for several hours until we insisted they go home to get some sleep. In the days that followed, family would surround us, friends would visit us and cook for us and we held Patrick's funeral six days after he died.

Months later, sitting there talking with Dr. Carol, I found that the source of my pain came from recalling finding Patrick that evening. It would come unbidden and jolt me like a cattle prod. And it made me anxious, nervous and short-tempered.

Dr. Carol suggested I look into a psychotherapy treatment called Accelerated Resolution Therapy (ART) which was originally created to help veterans suffering from PTSD. After doing research online, I found a local psychologist who is a Master ART Clinician and I met with her a couple times. I'm happy to report that those sessions were very beneficial to me, and I am much better now.

We should also check-in with ourselves occasionally. How do I react if someone shares with me that they are feeling depressed? Do I attempt to help them out? Listen to them? Comfort them?

Perhaps I shut down because it hurts too much to hear of their pain (this is my "go-to" move)? Or, do I argue with them that they are fine?

In Patrick's case that Wednesday evening, he went silent. I now believe that someone going silent is an early indication of a potential storm on the horizon. If someone we know or love goes silent, we should *check-in* with them to see how they are doing. Perhaps that reaching out might be what they need at the time to bring them back from the brink of disaster. Be supportive and encourage them to seek professional help if their situation has become dire. Engaging with a psychologist or psychiatrist might be what's best for them.

HOW

Assuming you have made it this far with me, and you're ready to take up the challenge to help others who are in pain, *how* do you even start? It might seem daunting, and you might fear that doing so will affect your relationship with the other person. I truly believe that we must take up the challenge because lives are in the balance, and doing nothing could hasten a horrible outcome.

I have suggested several ideas about *how* to start helping those dealing with mental health issues. The closing paragraph for many of the daily chapters includes those suggestions. Here are a few of them:

> From *Showing Up*:
>
> > I implore you to pay attention to how others are showing up with you.
>
> From *Denial*:
>
> > Stop denying what we see with our own eyes. Stop denying what we hear with our own ears. People in pain will often drop hints to us, perhaps subconsciously hoping that we will pick up on them and act upon them. They are crying out for help. We need to open our minds and our hearts to truly listen for their pleas. And don't fall prey to the stigma, where we turn away in denial. If we are open and don't deny what we see and hear:

Be receptive if they reach out to you.
Acknowledge their pain.
Help heal their pain.
Talk with them.
Comfort them.
Hold them.
Love them.

From *Salamander*:

It can be very difficult to find the emotional fortitude within ourselves that allows us to reach out and connect to someone who is in pain emotionally. Perhaps you are stronger than you think and you can help others in need. Have the courage to take the first step.

"You seem to be hurting. Can I help you?"

The most critical first steps to take aren't focused on another person, however. It starts with us being open to the possibility of being vulnerable with someone else, and being willing to get closer to them and understand their pain. Taking those first steps means you need to:

Open your eyes

Open your ears

Open your heart

Epilogue

DESTINATION

When I set out on this journey of the heart and mind, I didn't know in advance where it would take me. I was somewhat fearful of stirring up so many painful memories and I wasn't entirely sure that I would have the courage to complete what I had started. I wanted to believe that I had enough emotional fortitude to see it through to completion, but I did not know how the journey would affect me.

To be honest, I expected waterworks, most especially when I wrote the chapters entitled TRAGIC, CONSEQUENCES, PICK UP THE PIECES, RADIOACTIVE and CHECK-IN. And I especially enjoyed sharing the memories in Get Lost, The Wind, World Cup, Music and "Best Day of My Life."

The waterworks never came, and that surprised me. A lot. Perhaps that says something about how I've grown since my son's death. Or, it's more likely that I have my eye on the destination that is coming into focus as I reach the conclusion of my writing. The feedback I have received thus far from family and close friends has been encouraging, supportive and galvanizing at the same time. I'm starting to work out the details necessary for publishing this book and am hoping that it can reach as many people as possible.

I hope this makes a difference.

Please help me help others.

I pray that it be so.

About the Author

I know it's typical to include an *About the Author* section in a published book, but I have struggled looking at a blank page for several days now. That is because I am not a mental health professional. Who am I to provide advice about how to help others who have mental illness? My son died by suicide, so I obviously didn't help him enough. When I look in the mirror I see someone who ultimately failed his son. That is very hard to deal with at times, but life goes on and my family needs me.

What I have shared here has come from what I have experienced plus what I have surmised. I am not prescribing medication without a license, but I have provided advice based upon my awakening following my son's suicide.

Oh yeah, I'm supposed to use this page to share information about me, so I guess I better at least attempt to fulfill that obligation, so here goes…

> I'm a husband, father, son, brother, nephew, cousin, co-worker and a friend.
>
> I'm a Can-Am Spyder rider, and a race car driver/instructor.
>
> I have worked in the software industry for nearly four decades, in a variety of roles. I co-founded a start-up software company that was acquired eighteen months after we started it. My professional bio is on *LinkedIn*.

I am a first time author.

I am a public speaker and have done several "witnesses" at our church.

I am an amateur actor and have played Judas since 2013 in *The Living Last Supper* production that is performed at our church.

I was an associate producer and extra for the last four episodes of the award winning fan-produced series *Star Trek Continues.* I was also an associate producer and extra for the award winning fan-produced *Deadpool the Musical 2*.

And I'm damaged emotionally from the loss of my son.

Contact information:

Follow *Mind Crisis* on Facebook:
https://www.facebook.com/pathanavaniii

Appreciation

I would like to express my appreciation to the following people who have contributed to the journey I took while writing this book. They have either encouraged me, inspired me, validated or critiqued the book, provided edits or supported me emotionally during the journey:

My beloved wife, Lydia, and my cherished daughter, Christine. My parents, Pat Jr. and Alicia Hanavan. My best editor, my brother Mike Hanavan. My sisters, Theresa Vera and Cindy McElver. Lydia's sisters, Lea Donaldson, Mary Williams and Joy Adams. Brother-in-law, Pete Donaldson. My friend and neighbor, Mark McEwen. Dr. Laura Gallaher, Dr. Carol Mikulka, Dr. Angela Adams, Johnathon Thomas, Ashley Thomas and Gabriela Buich. Alice and Pat Viebey. Father John Bluett and Father Mike Roverse.

And special thanks to Father George Dunne whose kind words about a recent witness I did at our church re-ignited the spark in me to write this book.

Acknowledgements

All photographs Copyright © E. Patrick Hanavan III, except for those used by permission and annotated individually.

Harley Schwadron, *9 to 5* cartoon " I have this fear of the real world"
Copyright © 2019 Harley Schwadron

The Wind
Copyright © 1971 Cat Stevens, Island Records, a division of Universal Music Operations Limited

Always For You
Copyright © 2006 The Album Leaf, Sub Pop Records

Pick Up the Pieces
Copyright © 2018 Joe Bonamassa, J&R Adventures

Radioactive
Copyright © 2012 Imagine Dragons, KIDinaKORNER/Interscope Records

Pretty Fly (For a White Guy)
Copyright © 2016 The Offspring, Round Hill Records, Manufactured and distributed by Universal Music Enterprises, a division of UMG Recordings, Inc.

A Christmas Story
Copyright © 1983 Turner Entertainment Co., distributed by Warner

Made in the USA
Columbia, SC
16 February 2021

33059489R00083